High-Resolution CT
of the Chest

High-Resolution CT of the Chest

COMPREHENSIVE ATLAS

Eric J. Stern, M.D.

Assistant Professor of Radiology
Adjunct Assistant Professor of Medicine
University of Washington
Director of Thoracic Imaging
Harborview Medical Center
Seattle, Washington

Stephen J. Swensen, M.D.

Associate Professor of Radiology
Mayo Clinic
Rochester, Minnesota

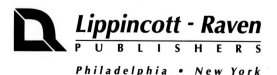

Lippincott - Raven
PUBLISHERS

Philadelphia • New York

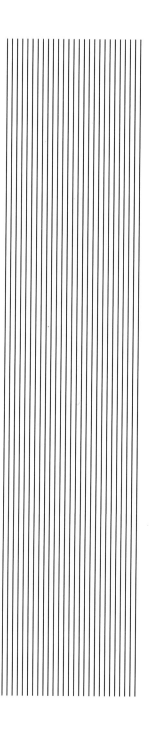

Acquisitions Editor: James D. Ryan
Sponsoring Editor: Susan R. Skand
Production Editor: Virginia Barishek
Production Manager: Janet Greenwood
Production: P. M. Gordon Associates, Inc.
Cover Designer: Becky Baxendell
Interior Designer: Arlene Putterman
Indexer: Dorothy Hoffman
Compositor: Pine Tree Composition
Prepress: Jay's Publishers Services
Printer/Binder: Quebecor/Kingsport

Library of Congress Cataloging-in-Publication Data

Stern, Eric J.
    High-resolution CT of the chest : comprehensive atlas / Eric J.
Stern, Stephen J. Swensen.
        p.   cm.
    Includes bibliographical references and index.
    ISBN 0–397–51451–4
    1. Chest—Tomography—Atlases.   I. Swensen, Stephen J.
II. Title.
    [DNLM: 1. Respiratory Tract Diseases—radiography—atlases.
2. Respiratory System—pathology—atlases.   3. Thoracic Radiography—
atlases.   4. Tomography, X-Ray Computed—atlases.   WF 17 S839h
1996]
RC941.S85   1996
617.5'407572—dc20
DNLM/DLC
for Library of Congress   95–44618
                                                              CIP

9   8   7   6   5   4   3   2   1

To my family, JES and EJS
and my mentors, WRW and GG
            —EJS

To Lynn
    —SJS

CONTRIBUTING
AUTHORS

Lisa Diethelm, M.D.
*Associate Professor of Radiology
Director, Thoracic and Cardiac Imaging
Louisiana State University Medical Center
New Orleans, Louisiana*

Georgeann Mcguinness, M.D.
*Assistant Professor of Radiology
New York University Medical Center
New York, New York*

Christopher J. Salmon, M.D.
*Assistant Professor of Radiology
Oregon Health Sciences University
Portland, Oregon*

Catherine A. Staples, M.D.
*Assistant Professor
Department of Radiology
University of British Columbia
St. Paul's Hospital
Vancouver, British Columbia, Canada*

ACKNOWLEDGMENTS

The authors and publisher wish to acknowledge the contribution of materials from the following sources:

Figures 3-2A, 3-8, 3-10, 3-12, 3-24, and 3-26 are reprinted with permission from: Stern EJ, Gamsu G. CT evaluation of airways diseases. The Radiologist 1994;1:335–344.

Figures 7-1, 7-2, 7-7, 7-13, 7-20, and 14-1 are reprinted with permission from: Stern EJ, Frank MS. CT of the lung in patients with pulmonary emphysema: Diagnosis, quantification, and correlation with pathologic and physiologic findings. AJR 1994;162:791–798.

Figures 2-14A, 3-11, 3-15, 3-20, 3-32, 3-34, 7-24, 7-27, 8-2, 10-3, 10-14, 11-17, 11-22, 11-23, and 13-24 are reprinted with permission from: Swensen SJ. Radiology of Thoracic Diseases. St. Louis: Mosby–Yearbook, 1993.

FOREWORD

As COAUTHOR of a textbook on high-resolution CT of the chest, it is a singular honor to be asked to write the foreword to an atlas on the same subject.

The aim of a reference textbook on high-resolution CT of the chest is to provide a thorough review of the literature and to illustrate the most common and characteristic features of diseases that affect the airways and pulmonary parenchyma. The aim of this atlas is to provide a pictorial essay of the spectrum of abnormalities that may be seen in any given disease entity. The textbook and the atlas therefore are complementary.

Optimal interpretation of any given image requires awareness of the underlying morphology and of the pathogenesis and evolution of the various disease processes. It also requires awareness that the manifestations of any disease process may be different in different patients or in different regions of lung in the same patient. The factors determining the high-resolution CT findings in any given disease entity are numerous, complex, and poorly understood. What is well recognized is that the high-resolution CT findings are influenced by the stage of the disease, whether predominantly inflammatory or fibrotic, by its severity, and by the presence of other concomitant processes.

Recognition of any given pattern of abnormality on high-resolution CT as being consistent with a certain disease or group of diseases is greatly facilitated by having previously seen the whole spectrum of findings. I congratulate the authors on their novel approach to the diagnosis of airway and parenchymal pulmonary disease.

Nestor L. Müller, M.D., Ph.D.

PREFACE

THIS COMPREHENSIVE ATLAS of high-resolution CT (HRCT) is in response to the often quoted statement that "diseases don't read the textbooks." This means that not every patient's disease process, confounded by a host of genetic and environmental factors, has a *classic* presentation of disease or presents at the same *stage* of disease as illustrated in the literature. Instead of showing one or two classic or typical appearances of a disease, this atlas is truer to "real life" situations and tries to include a spectrum of disease presentations, including the more unusual (the more typical?) presentations, i.e., very early or acute stages of a disease such as in lung fibrosis; the chronic or end-stages of a disease such as in pulmonary emphysema; atypical disease distributions such as with *Pneumocystis carinii* pneumonia; and mild and severe forms of a disease such as with bronchiectasis. In addition, to promote the understanding of the different manifestations and distributions of diseases within the lung, the spectrum of disease process within the same patient (e.g., comparing the upper lung zone appearance of eosinophilic granuloma with that in the middle and lower lung zones) is highlighted.

This book is intended primarily for the private radiology practitioner who has been hearing and reading about this technique called HRCT for the past few years and has begun to use it but finds that his or her images don't always look like previously published "classic" cases. In this atlas we have tried to group pathologic processes into similar groups, as found in the individual chapters. There are certain recognizable patterns of disease presentation and often a limited number of ways that different diseases can manifest within the lung; but like many other things in medicine, there is very little that is pathognomonic, even with HRCT. Many of the HRCT appearances we describe are relatively nonspecific, but when the images are interpreted in light of a specific clinical situation, often a very limited differential or specific diagnosis can be made.

Radiology residents-in-training would also benefit from an atlas of HRCT scanning that takes a spectrum of disease approach. Residents acquire their skills and radiologic acumen through seeing thousands of cases, almost all of which have at least slightly different appearances and clinical presentations. Residents need to see and integrate the many presentations of a disease; this atlas can help them achieve this goal.

The cases presented in this atlas include common abnormalities such as pulmonary emphysema and a variety of pulmonary infections that will appeal to clinical radiologists, as well as more unusual cases such as cystic lung disease and airways disease that will appeal to residents-in-training and those with a special interest in chest medicine.

HRCT scans represent the majority of cases shown in this book. However, to show the spectrum of certain disease presentations, some conventional CT scans of the chest are included as well.

Eric J. Stern, M.D.
Stephen J. Swensen, M.D.

CONTENTS

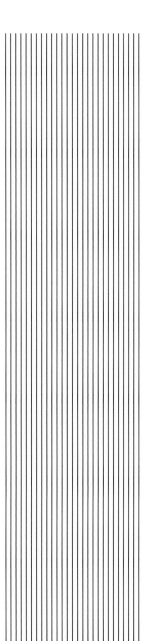

High-Resolution CT of the Chest: Comprehensive Atlas
by Eric J. Stern and Stephen J. Swensen,
Lippincott–Raven Publishers, Philadelphia © 1996.

Introduction to High-Resolution Computed Tomography

1

HIGH-RESOLUTION COMPUTED TOMOGRAPHY (HRCT) has contributed significantly to the radiologic assessment of intrathoracic disease in the last decade. The foremost reason is that HRCT scans detect and allow characterization of many disease processes that, in the conventional chest radiograph, are occult, nonspecific, or equivocal. For example, HRCT scans are particularly useful in diagnosing bronchiectasis, essentially making bronchography an obsolete examination.

TECHNIQUE

HRCT is a technique that can be performed on any late generation computed tomographic scanner. It differs from conventional computed tomography (CT) only in that it optimizes technical parameters for spatial resolution by using the narrowest beam collimation possible (usually 1 mm to 1.5 mm in diameter) and a high spatial frequency reconstruction algorithm (e.g., bone, sharp). Spatial resolution may be further increased by reducing the field of view to include just one lung, thereby effectively doubling the resolution. Narrowing the field of view is called targeting. This decreases the size of the pixels and therefore increases the spatial resolution. Targeting is generally not necessary to characterize most lung parenchymal disease processes.

Optimizing spatial resolution with HRCT usually means sacrificing complete cranial to caudal coverage of the lung; contiguous 1 mm scanning of the whole lung would require ≥300 slices. Although there is a role for HRCT in focal lung disease,[1,2] it should generally be considered a tool for sampling diffuse lung disease; for example, with 1 mm collimation, scans performed at 20 mm intervals show only 5% of the lung parenchyma as opposed to the 100% coverage obtained with conventional contiguous or spiral CT scanning. Actual HRCT scanning protocols vary somewhat from institution to institution and therefore we hesitate to recommend a single protocol; it is best to tailor the HRCT scan to the particular patient and clinical problem.

We suggest routine use of a single window/level combination (window level of about −750 Hounsfield units [HU] and a width of about 1500 HU), but we also recommend tailoring the window/level combination to accentuate certain disease processes. For instance, to increase confidence in detecting interstitial lung disease, we suggest using a window with higher contrast (window level of about −750 HU and a width of about 1000 to 1200 HU). For accentuating more subtle differences in lung density, such as in emphysema or obliterative bronchiolitis, a lower window level (−800 to −900 HU) and narrower width (500 to 1000 HU) increase the contrast between abnormal and normal lung tissue, although it must always be kept in mind that such a window can also make the normal interstitium appear abnormally prominent. Wider window widths of 1500 to 2000 HU reduce contrast between the lung and air-containing spaces but are useful for examining pleuroparenchymal abnormalities.

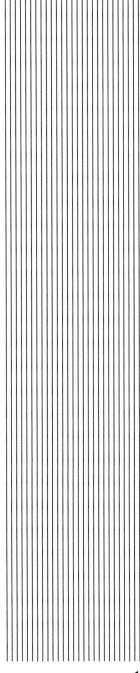

ANATOMY

HRCT scans can show lung anatomy and morphology not evident on conventional CT scans or plain radiographs. Because abnormalities are easily detected and characterized at the level of the secondary pulmonary lobule, it is important to have an understanding of the secondary lobule's anatomy, i.e., the intralobular core structures (the intralobular artery and airway) and the interlobular septa (containing the lobular venous and lymphatic drainage).

The acinus, the respiratory unit of the lung, is that portion of lung supplied by a terminal bronchiole and includes the gas-exchange structures (usually three to eight respiratory bronchioles, with subtending alveolar ducts and alveoli). Three to five acini form the secondary pulmonary lobule, or more simply, the pulmonary lobule. The acinus system of description is preferable for theoretical and functional reasons in some circumstances, whereas the lobular system is preferable in situations in which macroscopic tissue abnormalities are more important. The pulmonary acinus is not normally visible on HRCT (except in some disease states), whereas pulmonary lobular structures are well visualized on HRCT. Lobular terminology is important in radiologically defining many lung diseases, and it is used throughout this book.

PATTERNS OF DISEASE

In patients with infiltrative or diffuse lung disease, ground-glass opacity is a common but nonspecific HRCT finding.[3] Ground-glass attenuation is usually not evident on chest radiographs. Abnormalities that cause ground-glass opacities are beyond the limits of spatial resolution of HRCT and therefore appear as a generalized increase in the background density of the lung. The etiologies of ground-glass attenuation are numerous. Any process that decreases air content of the alveoli, or conversely that fills alveolar spaces or thickens interstitial structures, can produce ground-glass opacity, including inflammation and fibrosis. When ground-glass opacity is associated with lung architectural distortion, e.g., traction bronchiectasis, bronchiolectasis, or honeycombing, it is usually due to fibrosis. Although the finding of ground-glass attenuation is nonspecific, specific clinical settings help narrow the differential diagnostic possibilities, especially when anatomic distribution and any associated architectural abnormalities (or lack thereof) are also analyzed.

HRCT scans can identify small nodules not evident on chest radiographs. Small, rounded opacities on HRCT, especially poorly defined nodules, do not have to be "nodules" per se. They can be inflammatory or fibrotic regions of lung, around small bronchovascular bundles, that only appear as nodules, e.g., with hypersensitivity pneumonitis. The lumina of small airways may be obliterated, thereby making them appear as nodules, e.g., as occurs in panbronchiolitis and cystic fibrosis.

Especially in the early stages of lung damage, HRCT is more sensitive and accurate than either chest radiographs or pulmonary function tests in defining the presence and extent of both pulmonary emphysema[4] and cystic lung diseases[5] in symptomatic patients. In cystic lung diseases, HRCT separates out the superimposition of multiple thin walls of lung cysts responsible for the interstitial pattern observed on chest radiography, accurately displaying the extent and distribution of cystic change of the lung. Also, HRCT better displays the individual cystic walls than routine 8 mm to 10 mm section CT.

HRCT is also more sensitive than chest radiography or conventional CT scanning for detecting lung and pleural abnormalities in asbestos-exposed individuals. HRCT is helpful in eliminating false-positive chest radiographic diagnoses of asbestos-related pleural disease caused by subpleural fat and false-positive diagnoses of asbestosis in patients with extensive pleural plaques or superimposed emphysema.[6]

CT and HRCT have been shown to be very useful in the evaluation of focal lung disease.[1,2] HRCT is more sensitive than CT and chest radiography in the detection of fat and calcium in lung nodules. HRCT often allows a confident, specific diagnosis of a benign process to be made, such as granuloma, hamartoma, rounded atelectasis, arteriovenous malformation, and extralobar bronchopulmonary sequestration, thus obviating the need for invasive diagnostic procedures and saving patient expense and morbidity. In general, focal lung disease is best initially localized with conventional CT, usually of the entire thorax to determine if a lung lesion is solitary. HRCT scans can then be selectively obtained, depending on the CT appearance and clinical situation.

HRCT scanning is useful in examining the lungs in patients who have fevers or respiratory symptoms but normal or nonspecific chest radiographs, again by detecting, characterizing, and localizing disease. For example, HRCT scanning can assess the severity of disease in patients with bronchiectasis and cystic fibrosis[7] or identify active granulomatous disease in patients with prior mycobacterial infection.[8]

CT and especially HRCT scans obtained at suspended full expiration in patients with fixed or reactive small airways diseases take advantage of air trapping, accentuating subtle differences in lung attenuation between normal and abnormal lung parenchyma. Air trapping has been shown in asthmatics,[9] in obliterative bronchiolitis[10] of all etiologies (including the postinfectious Swyer-James syndrome[11]), and in cystic fibrosis.[12] Expiratory CT scanning provides both anatomic and physiologic information that is complementary to both conventional suspended full-inspiration CT and pulmonary function testing. Depending on the clinical scenario, knowing the extent and distribution of air trapping is useful in indicating or directing further diagnostic work-up, such as transbronchial, thoracoscopic, or open lung biopsy.

REFERENCES

1. Webb WR. Radiologic evaluation of the solitary pulmonary nodule. AJR 1990; 154: 701–708

2. Swensen SJ. Focal lung disease: CT and high-resolution CT applications. Radiographics 1994; 14:169–181

3. Engeler CE, Tashjian JH, Trenkner SW, Walsh JW. Ground-glass opacity of the lung parenchyma: A guide to analysis with high-resolution CT. AJR 1993; 160:249–251

4. Klein JS, Gamsu G, Webb WR, Golden JA, Müller NL. High-resolution CT diagnosis of emphysema in symptomatic patients with normal chest radiographs and isolated low diffusing capacity. Radiology 1992; 182:817–821

5. Stern EJ, Webb WR, Golden JA, Gamsu G. Cystic lung disease associated with eosinophilic granuloma and tuberous sclerosis: Air trapping at dynamic ultrafast high-resolution CT. Radiology 1992; 182:325–329

6. Friedman AC, Fiel SB, Fisher MS, Radecki PD, Lev TA, Caroline DF. Asbestos-related pleural disease and asbestosis: A comparison of CT and chest radiography. AJR 1988; 150:269–275

7. Kuhn JP. High-resolution computed tomography of pediatric pulmonary parenchymal disorders. Radiol Clin North Am 1993; 31:533–551

8. Im JG, Itoh H, Shim YS, et al. Pulmonary tuberculosis: CT Findings—early active disease and sequential change with antituberculous therapy. Radiology 1993; 186:653–660

9. Stern EJ, Frank MS. Small-airway diseases of the lungs: Findings at expiratory CT. AJR 1994; 163:37–41

10. Sweatman MC, Millar AB, Strickland B, Turner WM. Computed tomography in adult obliterative bronchiolitis. Clin Radiol 1990; 41:116–119

11. Moore AD, Godwin JD, Dietrich PA, Verschakelen JA, Henderson WRJ. Swyer-James syndrome: CT findings in eight patients. AJR 1992; 158:1211–1215

12. Lynch DA, Brasch RC, Hardy KA, Webb WR. Pediatric pulmonary disease: Assessment with high-resolution ultrafast CT. Radiology 1990; 176:243–248

High-Resolution CT of the Chest: Comprehensive Atlas
by Eric J. Stern and Stephen J. Swensen,
Lippincott–Raven Publishers, Philadelphia © 1996.

Anatomy
2

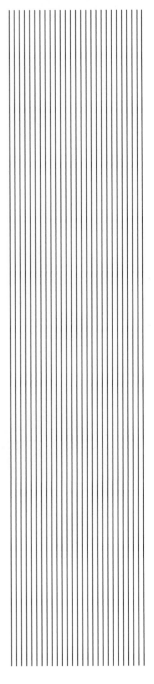

NORMAL APPEARANCE OF THE AIRWAYS, VESSELS, AND FISSURES
Normal tracheal anatomy

INSPIRATION

EXPIRATION

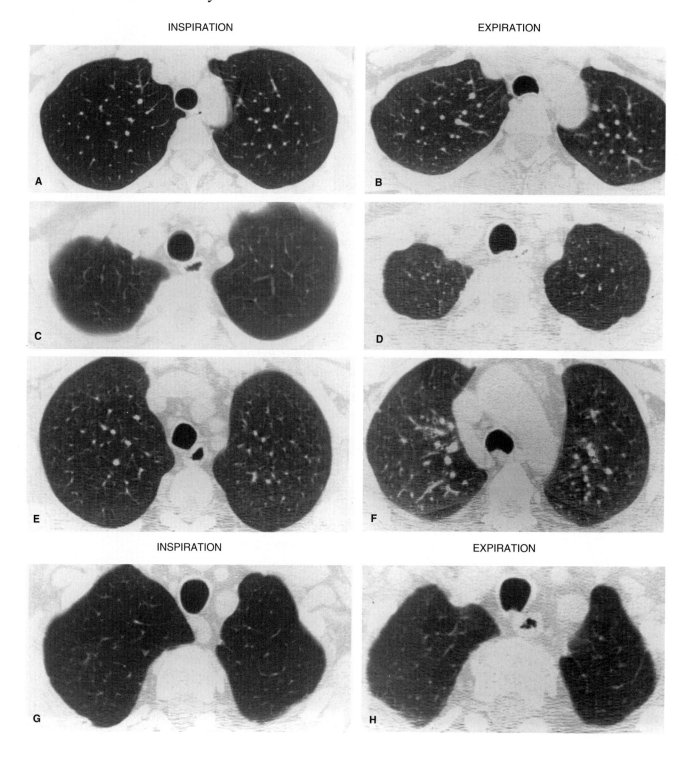

INSPIRATION

EXPIRATION

FIGURE 2-1

CT scans through the trachea in four different patients, performed at both suspended full inspiration and expiration, show slight differences in the tracheal contours among patients. The trachea is usually round or nearly round at inspiration. The coronal-sagittal diameter ratio is approximately 1:1. At expiration the posterior membrane moves anteriorly, giving the trachea an inverted U shape. The cross-sectional area of the trachea should not decrease more than 60% at end-expiration.[1]

Normal bronchial cartilages

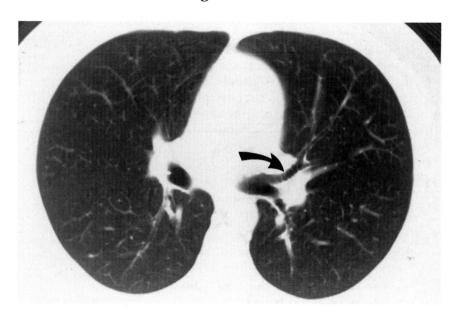

FIGURE 2-2
HRCT scan shows the bronchial cartilage rings in the left upper lobe bronchus (*arrow*). This is a normal finding.

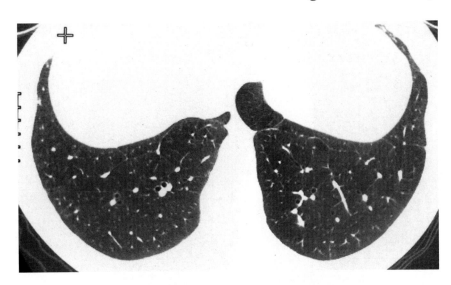

FIGURE 2-3

HRCT scan shows normal subsegmental bronchial airways in both lower lobes. Compare the size of the airway to its accompanying artery in the bronchovascular bundles. Note the barely perceptible thickness of the normal airway wall.

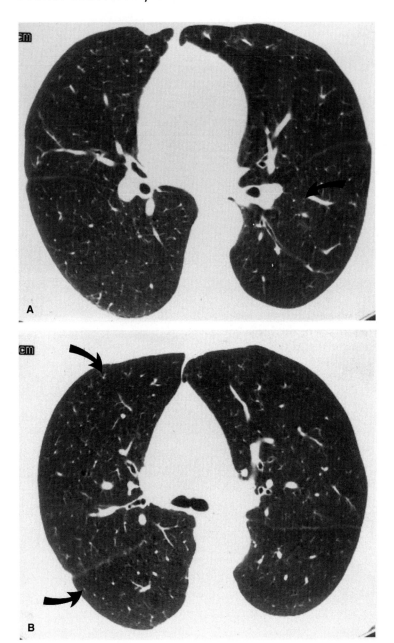

FIGURE 2-4

(A) With optimal scanning technique, HRCT can routinely image airways to approximately their eighth generation branches (*arrow*). Normal airways are therefore not detectable in the peripheral half of the lung. Pulmonary arteries may be imaged out to approximately 16th generation branches. (B) This allows imaging of lobular bronchiolar arteries to within 5 mm to 10 mm of the pleura, often with a typical V shape, separated by 1 to 2 cm (*arrows*). Note that the accompanying intralobular bronchiole is not visualized at this level.

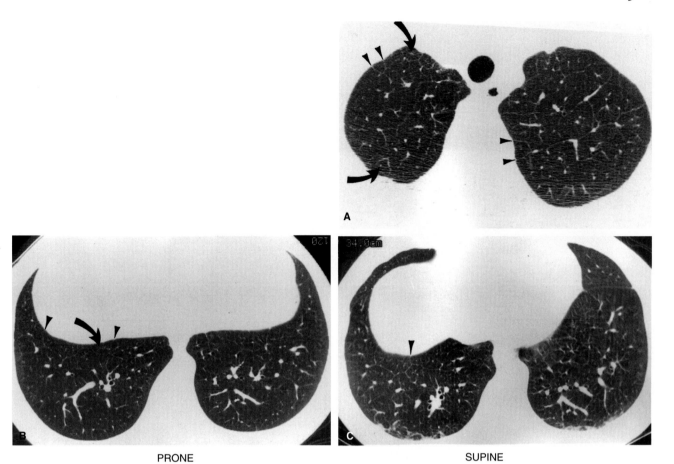

PRONE   SUPINE

FIGURE 2-5

HRCT scans can show normal lung anatomic and morphologic features that cannot be obtained using conventional CT or plain radiographs. Since abnormalities are easily detected at the level of the secondary pulmonary lobule, it is important to have an understanding of normal secondary pulmonary lobular structures and their normal appearance. Of the centrilobular core structures, only the centrilobular artery can normally be visualized (*arrows*); the centrilobular bronchiole is never seen in healthy individuals. The secondary pulmonary lobules are separated by interlobular septa that are not normally visible on HRCT, except as an occasional thin line at the extreme periphery of the lung, usually at the lung bases (*arrowheads*). The interlobular septa contain venules and lymphatics that drain the secondary pulmonary lobules. Certain pathologic processes, which usually involve the lymphatics, accentuate or thicken the interlobular septa, making them visible by HRCT (see Figs. 2-14 to 2-23).

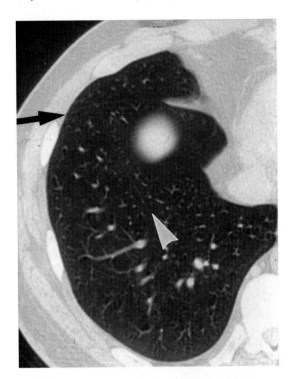

FIGURE 2-6

HRCT scan shows right major (*arrow*) and inferior accessory (*arrowhead*) fissures. The inferior accessory fissure separates the medial basal segment from the other basilar segments. Accessory fissures are present in approximately 3% to 5% of the population.

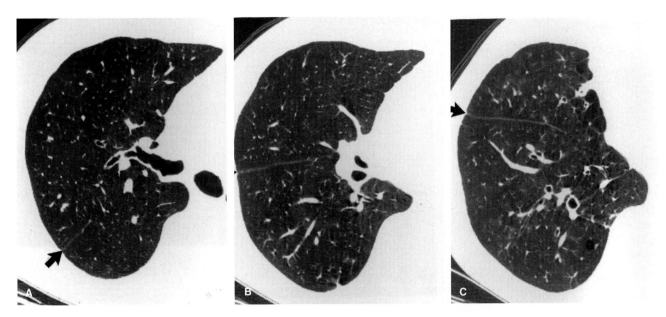

FIGURE 2-7

HRCT scans show an incomplete interlobar fissure (*arrow*) as a discontinuous linear opacity that remains in contact with the chest wall. Bronchovascular structures cross through the two fused lobes. This is a common finding that may be seen in up to 80% of individuals and should not be misinterpreted as a linear scar or atelectasis.[2] Recognition of an incomplete interlobar fissure is occasionally important in understanding the spread of pulmonary disease or in explaining various patterns of collapse or lack thereof in obstructed airways.

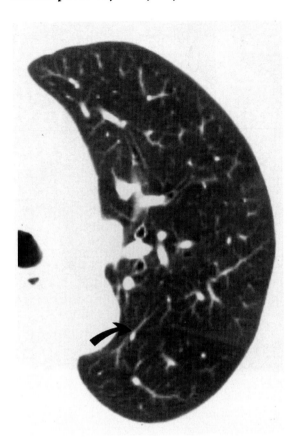

FIGURE 2-8

HRCT scan again shows an incomplete interlobar fissure as a discontinuous linear opacity that remains in contact with the chest wall. Note the small pulmonary artery crossing through the fused portion of the lung (*arrow*).

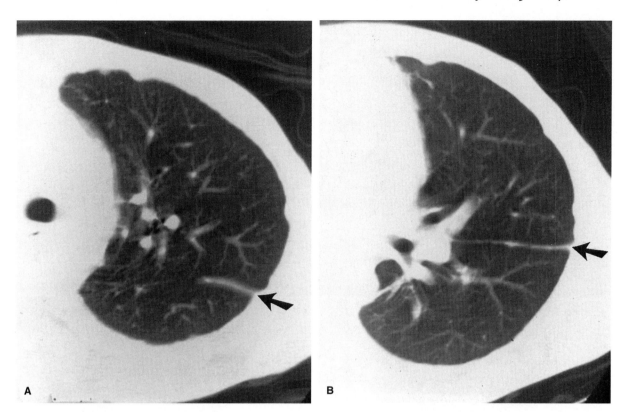

FIGURE 2-9

CT scans in this patient with a left tuberculous pleural effusion show both an incomplete major fissure (*arrow*) (A) and a complete major fissure (*arrow*) (B) at a more caudal level.

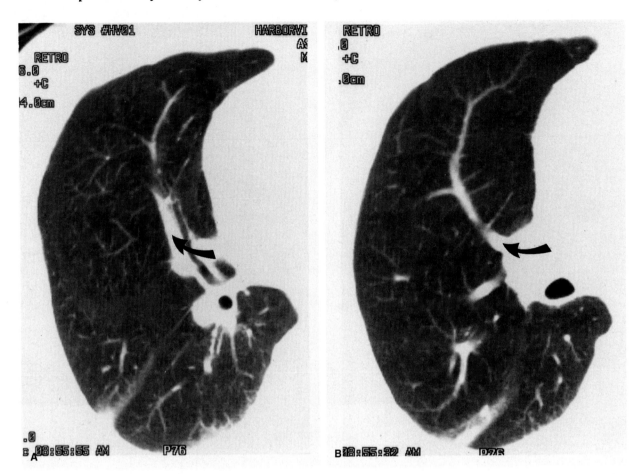

FIGURE 2-10

Consecutive 3 mm CT scans through the right hilum show the middle pulmonary artery (*arrow*) and bronchus (A) traveling together in the bronchovascular bundle; they show a dichotomous branching pattern, the branches arising at acute angles. The middle lobe vein (*arrow*) (B), like all pulmonary veins, has a monopodal branching pattern; the branches arise at approximately 90-degree angles, with no accompanying airway.

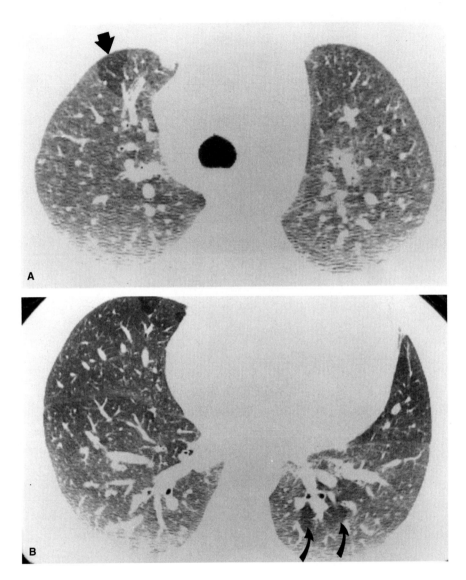

FIGURE 2-11

HRCT scans obtained at suspended end-expiration show several hyperlucent secondary pulmonary lobules outlined by normal lung (*arrows*). The secondary pulmonary lobules are seen because of air trapping in this patient with asthma. Note the small white dots—the centrilobular core structures—at the center of the lucencies.

Secondary pulmonary lobule

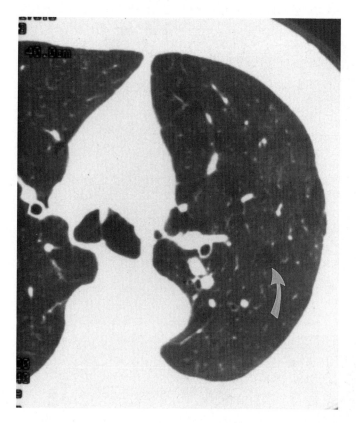

FIGURE 2-12

HRCT scan in this patient with pneumonia shows a normal secondary pulmonary lobule (*arrow*) outlined by ground-glass opacity in adjacent lobules. This normally aerated pulmonary lobule is spared, at least for the moment, from the surrounding pneumonitis. Again note the small white dots—the centrilobular core structure—at the center of the lucencies.

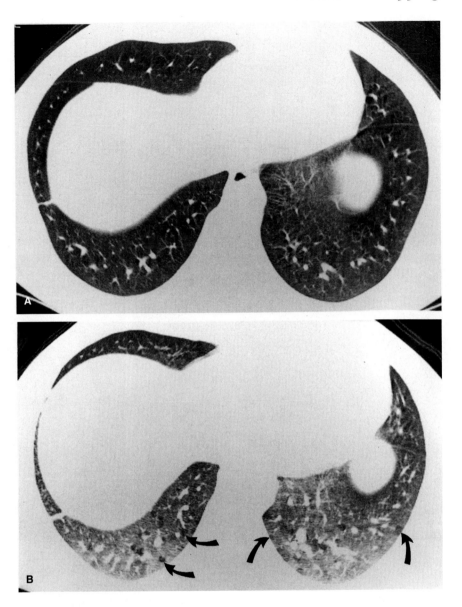

FIGURE 2-13

HRCT scan in this patient with acquired immunodeficiency syndrome (AIDS) and chronic cough, obtained at suspended end-inspiration (*left*), is normal. HRCT scan obtained at suspended end-expiration (*right*) at the same level as in (A) shows multiple acinar-sized hyperlucencies (*arrows*) outlined by normal lung in this patient with presumptive bronchiolitis. Again, note the small white dots—the centriacinar core structures—at the center of the lucencies.

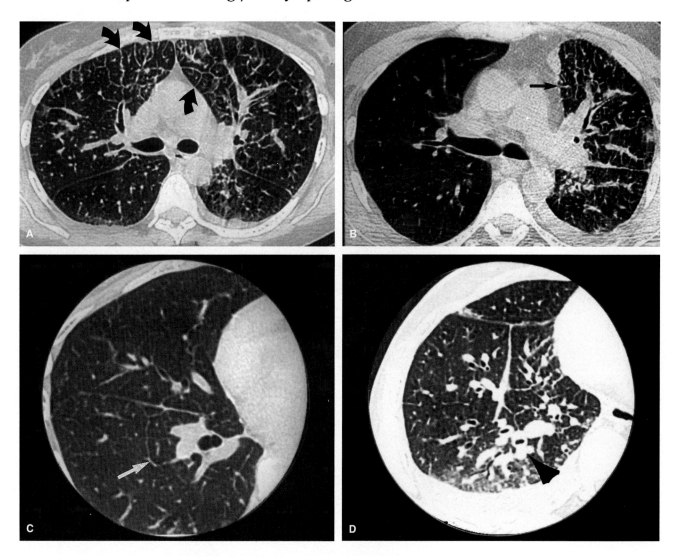

FIGURE 2-14

HRCT scans from four different patients show characteristic findings of lymphangitic carcinomatosis. Note both nodular and smooth interlobular septal thickening (*arrows*). Also note the thickened fissures, probably from subpleural lymphatic involvement. There is also thickening of the bronchovascular bundle (*arrowheads*). In this disease, there is a combination of tumor cell infiltration and lymphatic obstruction in the interstitial space.

Thickened septa are a nonspecific finding and may represent thickening from edema, cellular infiltration, or fibrosis. Lymphangitic carcinomatosis often shows a nodular or irregular thickening of the septa without the anatomic distortion of pulmonary fibrosis or the smooth thickening of edema. In this disease, tumor cells infiltrate and thicken the interstitium and obstruct the lymphatic channels.

Sarcoidosis may resemble lymphangitic carcinomatosis. In general, sarcoidosis tends to be more central, perihilar, and symmetrically bilateral in its distribution.

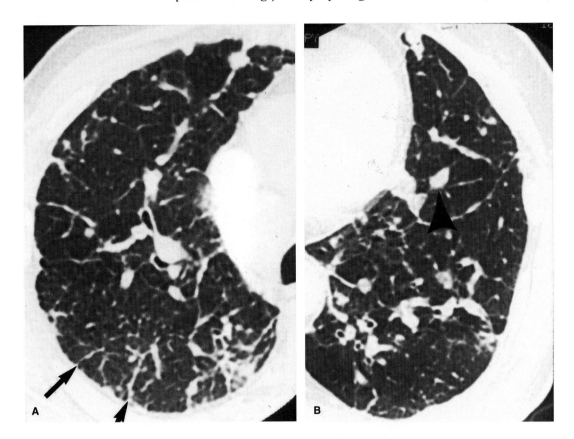

FIGURE 2-15

HRCT scans show two different appearances of lymphangitic carcinomatosis in the same patient. The distribution of disease in the left lung has a prominent axial (central) distribution (*arrowhead*), with thickened bronchovascular bundles. There is a more peripheral distribution (septal lines) in the right lung.

Minimal interlobular septal thickening from lymphangitic carcinomatosis

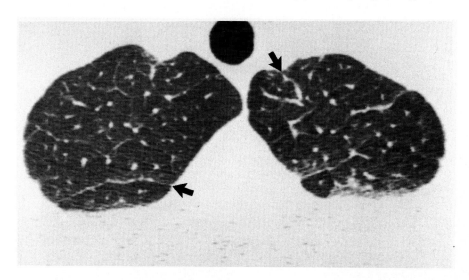

FIGURE 2-16

HRCT scan shows minimal, somewhat beaded, interlobular septal thickening (*arrows*) in early lymphangitic carcinomatosis.

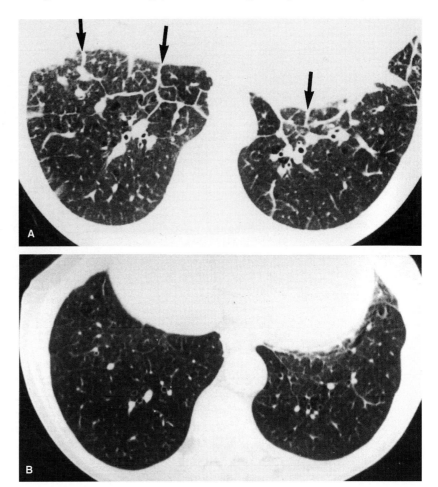

FIGURE 2-17

HRCT scans performed at the same anatomic level before and after medical therapy for cardiogenic pulmonary edema show resolution of the thickened interlobular septa in (A) (*arrows*). In this patient, distention of lymphatic channels and interstitial edema secondary to elevated left ventricular end-diastolic pressure resulted in thickened interlobular septa. These structures represent the Kerley B lines seen on chest radiographs. This case illustrates the nonspecific nature of visible, thickened septa.

Cardiogenic pulmonary edema

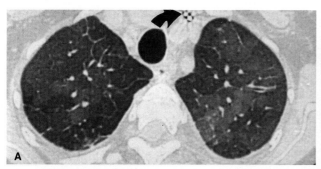
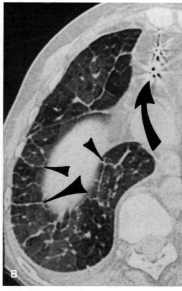

FIGURE 2-18

HRCT scans show ground-glass opacification throughout the lungs, with patchy sparing of many secondary pulmonary lobules. There is moderately smooth thickening of the interlobular septa, most marked in the bases (*arrowheads*). Also present were small bilateral pleural effusions, not included on these images. Note star artifacts from transvenous cardiac pacemaker (*curved arrows*). These HRCT findings are characteristic of cardiogenic pulmonary edema, either related to primary elevation of left atrial pressure such as with mitral stenosis or mitral regurgitation or related to elevated left ventricular end-diastolic pressure such as with dilated or restrictive cardiomyopathy.

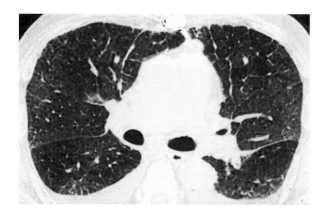

FIGURE 2-19

HRCT scan shows diffuse bilateral infiltrates that have a predominantly basilar distribution. Also present are ground-glass opacities, mild smooth thickening of interlobular septa and the major fissures, and mild peribronchovascular thickening. These findings are most compatible with and in this case were caused by pulmonary edema from dysfunction of the left ventricular myocardium.

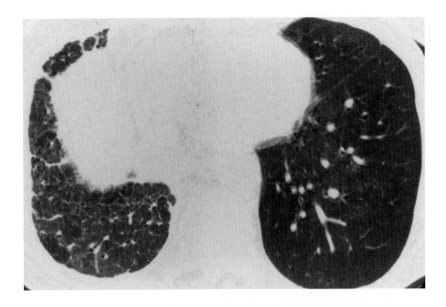

FIGURE 2-20

HRCT scan after right lung transplantation for emphysema shows smooth thickening of ipsilateral peripheral interlobular septa due to pulmonary lymphatic disruption.

Interlobular septal thickening from a resolving pneumonia

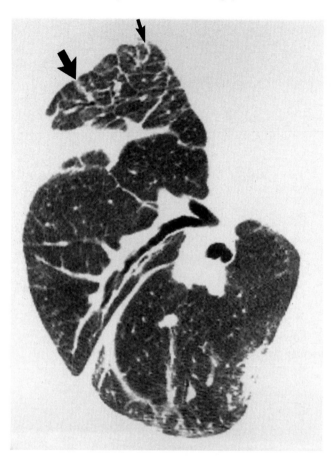

FIGURE 2-21

HRCT scan in this patient with a resolving pneumonia shows thickened and distorted septa (*arrows*). After an insult, the lung heals by draining exudates and edema through the lymphatic channels. This may cause the lymphatics to appear prominent, as in this case.

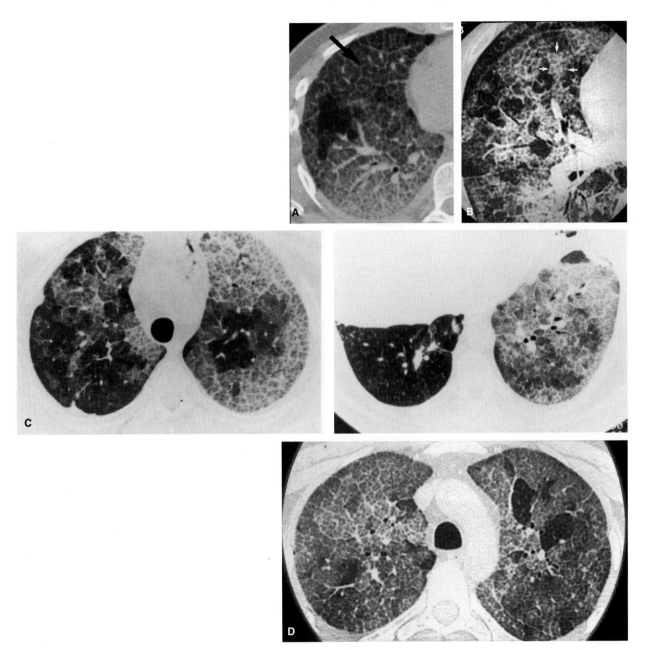

FIGURE 2-22

HRCT scans from four patients with alveolar proteinosis. Note the thickened interlobular septa and intralobular structures, many of which have a typical polygonal shape (*black arrow*).

Alveolar proteinosis has both interstitial and air space components. The groundglass opacification of alveolar spaces (*white arrows*) reflects the presence of phospholipid/proteinaceous material in them. The same material is incorporated into the interstitium with consequent thickening of the interlobular septa, an HRCT finding not appreciable on chest radiographs. This combination of HRCT findings is typical for this disease, although sarcoidosis and *pneumocystis carinii* pneumonia can have a similar appearance (see Figs. 11-9 through 11-11 and Fig. 13-9).

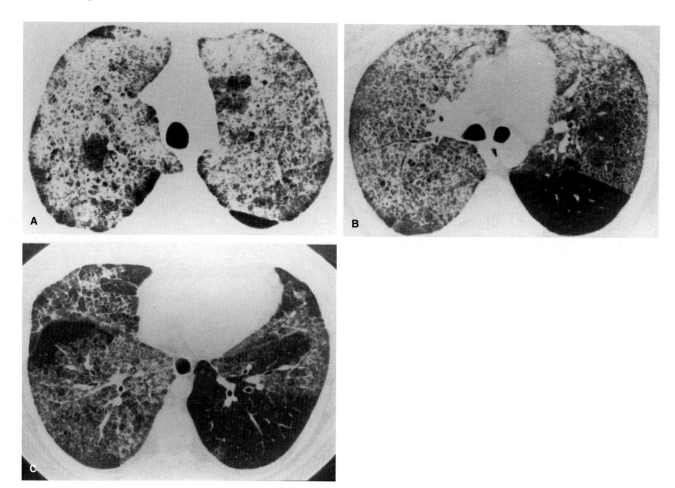

FIGURE 2-23
HRCT scans show the patchy distribution of disease that may occur with alveolar proteinosis.

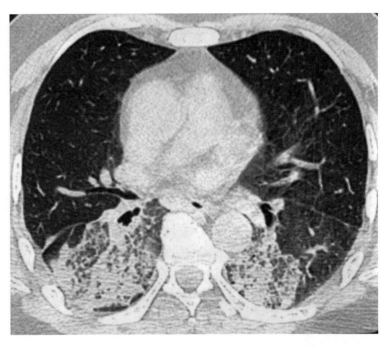

FIGURE 2-24

HRCT scan shows an atypical posterior-basal distribution in this case of alveolar proteinosis, probably secondary to exogenous lipid pneumonia.

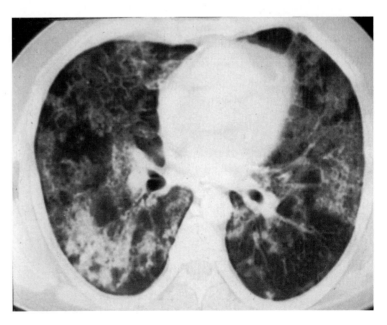

FIGURE 2-25

CT scan shows another atypical case of alveolar proteinosis. Note that there is less "crazy-paving" and more homogeneous opacification.

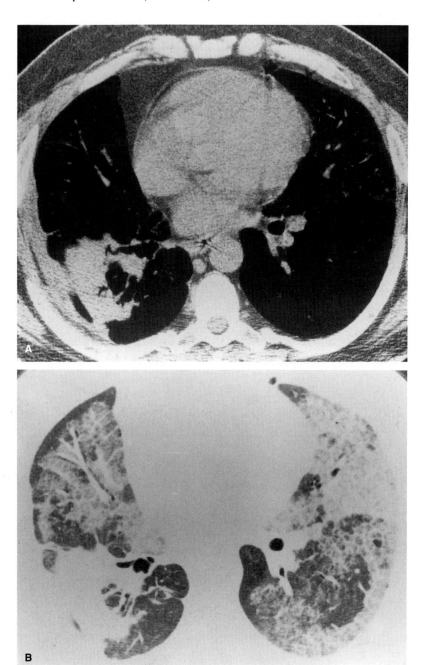

FIGURE 2-26

HRCT scans in this patient with alveolar proteinosis show an area of confluent, well-demarcated opacification in the lateral basal segment of the right lower lobe as a new focal finding. This was caused by a secondary infection with *Nocardia,* not an infrequent complication of alveolar proteinosis.

REFERENCES

1. Stern EJ, Graham CM, Webb WR, Gamsu G. Normal trachea during forced expiration: Dynamic CT measurements. Radiology 1993; 187:27–31

2. Otsuji H, Uchida H, Maeda M, et al. Incomplete interlobar fissures: Bronchovascular analysis with CT. Radiology 1993; 187:541–546

High-Resolution CT of the Chest: Comprehensive Atlas
by Eric J. Stern and Stephen J. Swensen,
Lippincott–Raven Publishers, Philadelphia © 1996.

Large Airways Diseases

3

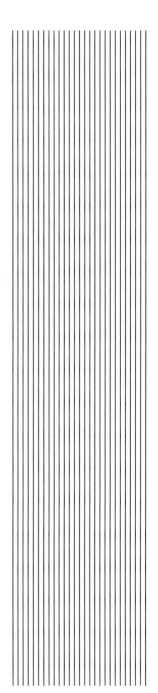

Tracheobronchomegaly (Mounier-Kuhn syndrome)

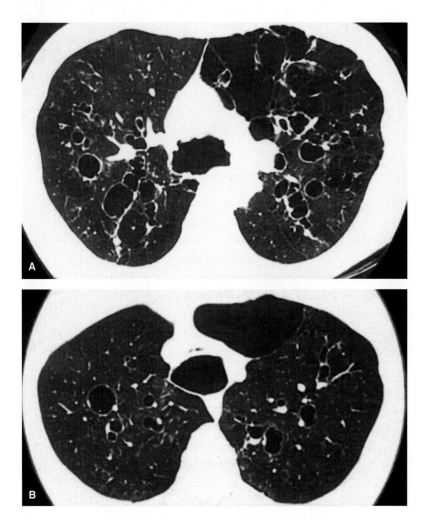

FIGURE 3-1

HRCT scans show typical findings of tracheobronchomegaly (TBM). Note marked tracheal enlargement (>30 mm in this patient; normal is <25 mm) and extensive central bronchiectasis bilaterally. The typical CT features of TBM are dilatation of the trachea and mainstem bronchi, tracheal diverticulosis, bronchiectasis, and chronic pulmonary parenchymal disease.[1] Tracheal disorders can be categorized as diffuse or focal abnormalities. Although some of these tracheal abnormalities are fairly common, most are very uncommon.

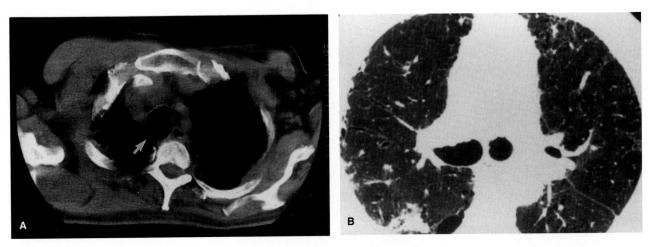

FIGURE 3-2

HRCT scan from a patient with TBM shows an associated tracheal diverticulum (*arrow* in A). The bronchus intermedius is dilated to the size of a normal trachea. Note the mild peripheral bronchiectasis and chronic parenchymal scarring, in (B).

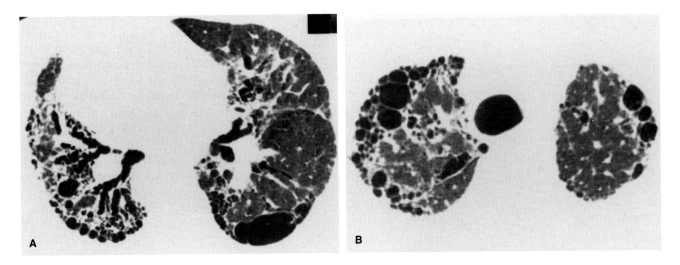

FIGURE 3-3

HRCT scans show severe cystic bronchiectasis and parenchymal scarring (A) associated with the TBM (32 mm tracheal diameter in B). TBM is a rare disorder, probably congenital in origin. The diagnosis is made radiologically.[2] Although TBM may be suggested on chest radiographs, CT has been used to confirm the diagnosis.

Saber sheath tracheal deformity

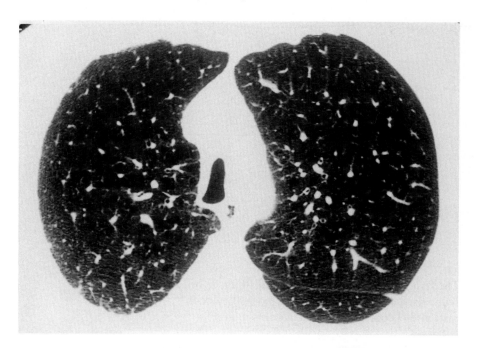

FIGURE 3-4

HRCT scan shows a typical severe saber sheath tracheal deformity commonly found in conjunction with chronic bronchitis and chronic obstructive pulmonary disease.[3] Because this abnormality reflects the influence of chronically increased intrathoracic pressures, probably from chronic coughing, the characteristic deformity involves only the intrathoracic trachea. The trachea is usually round or elliptical in cross-section (see Fig. 2-1); however, in saber sheath deformity the sagittal dimension is often twice the coronal dimension or greater.

The trachea and main bronchi may be decreased in caliber. Specific disease processes include tracheomalacia, saber sheath deformity, amyloidosis (primary and secondary types), relapsing polychondritis, tracheobronchopathia osteochondroplastica, and complete cartilage rings (also called napkin ring anomaly or congenital tracheal stenosis).

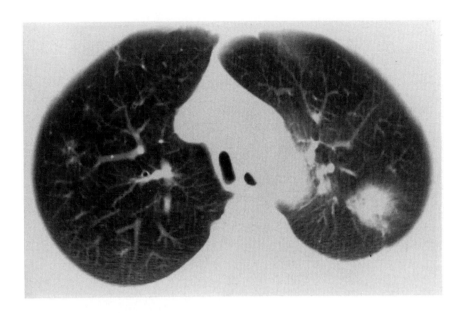

FIGURE 3-5

HRCT scan shows a severe saber sheath deformity of the intrathoracic trachea and an associated left lung cancer; both findings probably resulted from the effects of cigarette smoking.

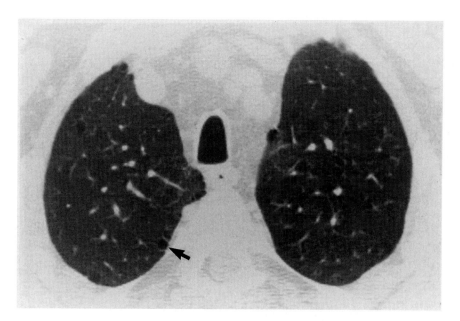

FIGURE 3-6

HRCT scan shows a mild saber sheath tracheal deformity with less coronal narrowing and only limited sagittal increase. Note the mild paraseptal emphysema (*arrow*; see Fig. 7-20).

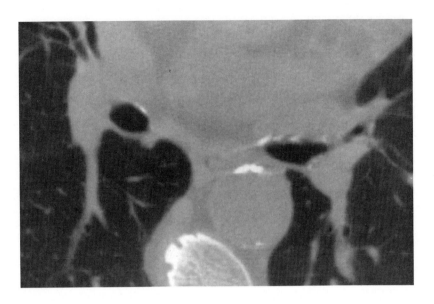

FIGURE 3-7

HRCT scan shows smooth, thin calcification of the walls of the main bronchi, with no intraluminal encroachment. This is usually an incidental finding, especially with advancing patient age.

Central airway amyloidosis

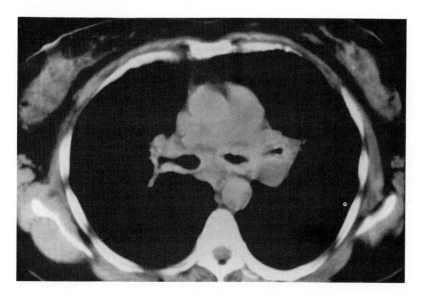

FIGURE 3-8

CT scan shows irregular thickening and calcification of the walls of the main bronchi. In amyloidosis, deposition of a protein-polysaccharide complex occurs in the submucosa and muscular layers of the airways. This forms irregular lardlike masses that are circumferential and encroach upon the airway lumen, narrowing it. This may be a focal or diffuse process and occurs as a primary or secondary abnormality.

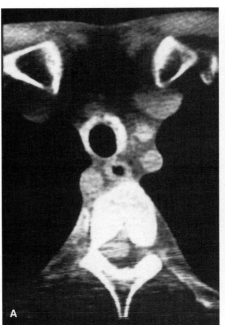 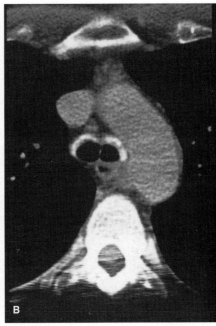

FIGURE 3-9

CT scans show thickening of the tracheal and mainstem bronchial walls with diffuse calcification that spares the posterior airway. These findings were caused by relapsing polychondritis. Differential diagnostic considerations include amyloidosis, tracheopathia osteochondroplastica, and Wegener's granulomatosis. Relapsing polychondritis is an unusual, idiopathic inflammatory systemic disease that affects the cartilage at many sites, including the ears, nose, joints, and tracheobronchial cartilages. Relapsing polychondritis causes a diffuse or focal fixed narrowing of the airway that is shown well on CT. The CT findings include diffuse, smooth tracheobronchial wall thickening with narrowing and deformity of the lumen. There may be dense calcium deposition within the thickened tracheal cartilages. These findings may diminish or return to normal after steroid therapy.[4]

Tracheobronchopathia osteochondroplastica

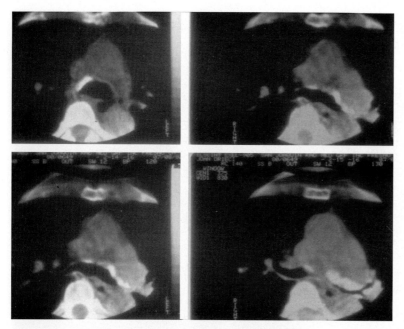

Figure 3-10

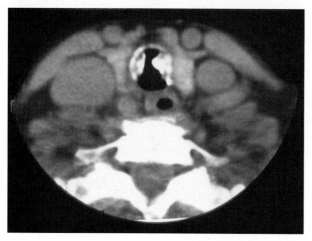

Figure 3-11

FIGURES 3-10 and 3-11

CT scans show characteristic findings of tracheopathia osteochondroplastica: calcified tracheal cartilaginous ring with nodular calcific protuberances that narrow the lumen. Tracheobronchopathia osteochondroplastica is an unusual idiopathic condition of unknown origin in which nodules of mature bone, bone marrow, and cartilage form and protrude into the lumen of the airway, usually the trachea, but with subglottic sparing. It is most common in men >50 years old and is usually asymptomatic. The incidence is reported as 1/200 in autopsy series; 90% of cases are diagnosed at autopsy as an incidental finding, although some patients may present during life with hemoptysis, usually due to mucosal erosion. Most cases, however, cause no symptoms and are only diagnosed incidentally during intubation or endoscopy. The diagnosis is usually made by endoscopy or CT scan. The CT appearance is similar to that of amyloidosis except that there is sparing of the posterior membrane; this process primarily affects the cartilage rings.

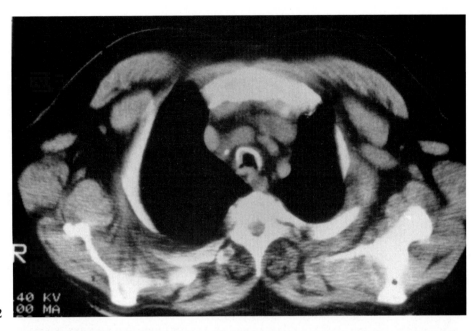

Figure 3-12

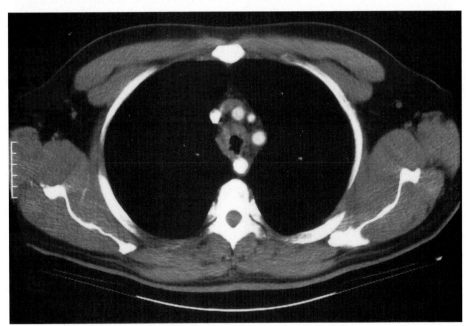

Figure 3-13

FIGURES 3-12 and 3-13

In Figure 3-12, the CT scan shows circumferential narrowing of the midtrachea due to inflammatory granulomata. In Figure 3-13, in addition to narrowing, the CT scan shows diffuse thickening of the tracheal wall. The tracheal narrowing in these two patients was caused by Wegener's granulomatosis. Other etiologies that yield similar CT findings include trauma tuberculosis, fungal infection, and laryngeal papillomatosis. CT is useful in ruling out extrinsic compression of the trachea by a mass or vascular anomaly. Other CT features of Wegener's granulomatosis involving the lung are found in Figures 10-24, 10-25, 10-26, and 10-27.

Adenoid cystic carcinoma

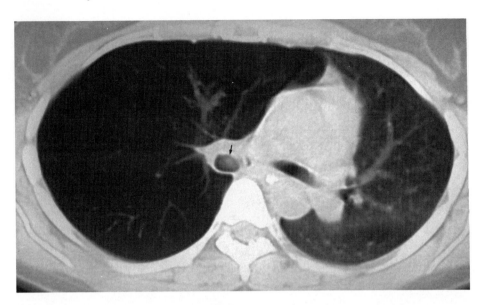

FIGURE 3-14

CT scan shows a right mainstem endobronchial lesion that was subsequently shown to be an adenoid cystic carcinoma, also called a cylindroma (*arrow*). This expiratory CT shows significant shift of the mediastinum to the left because of air trapping by the right lung with normal left lung deflation.

Benign neoplasms of the trachea are uncommon. They include chondromatous hamartoma, squamous cell papilloma, hemangioma, granular cell myoblastoma, leiomyoma, and other mesenchymal tumors. Squamous cell papillomas arise from human papilloma virus infection disseminated from the larynx to the trachea; they are most often seen in children and are usually multiple. The papilloma virus may also spread into the lung parenchyma—especially after instrumentation—where it causes multiple cavitating nodules, usually in a dependent distribution. Rarely, squamous cell papillomas undergo malignant transformation.

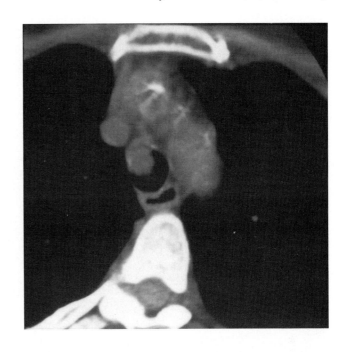

FIGURE 3-15

CT scan shows a 12 mm lesion arising from the anterior wall of the midtrachea. Diagnosis was adenoid cystic carcinoma (cylindroma).

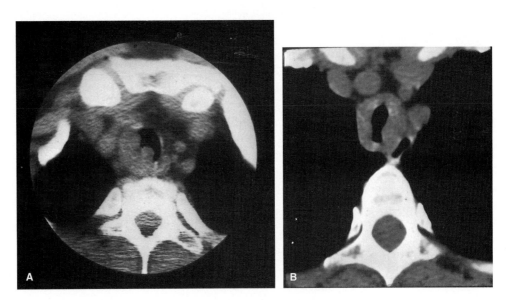

FIGURE 3-16

CT scan in (A) shows a lobulated mass arising from the right posterior and lateral aspects of the trachea and in (B) shows circumferential thickening of the wall of the trachea, both typical of infiltrative neoplasms, in these examples of adenoid cystic carcinoma. Differential diagnostic considerations would include squamous cell carcinoma, papilloma, chondrosarcoma, mucoepidermoid tumor, carcinoid tumor, and metastasis.

Leiomyoma

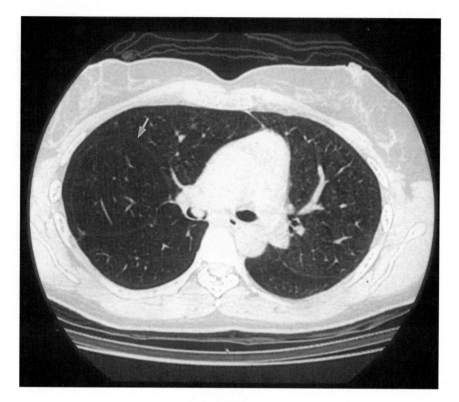

FIGURE 3-17

HRCT scan shows an endobronchial lesion nearly completely filling the bronchus intermedius just below the origin of the right upper lobe bronchus. Note the hyperlucent and hyperexpanded right lung as a result of air trapping. The diagnosis was benign leiomyoma. Note the HRCT appearance of a minor fissure (*arrow*).

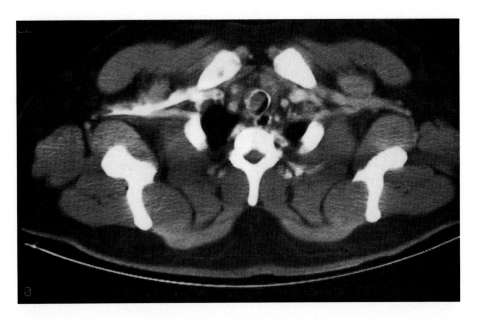

FIGURE 3-18

CT scan shows a 1.5 cm tracheal nodule extending from the right lateral wall. This
was a chondrosarcoma arising from one of the tracheal cartilage rings.

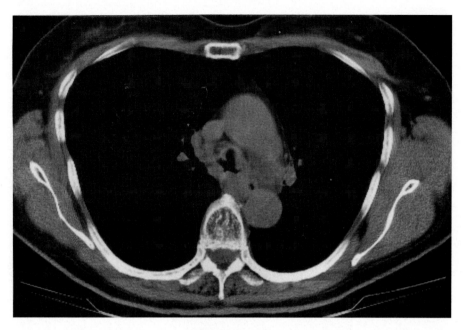

FIGURE 3-19

CT scan shows an irregular, lobular mass involving the posterior wall of the lower intrathoracic trachea. There is a large posterior, extraluminal component as well. The diagnosis was tracheal squamous cell carcinoma.

Primary malignant tracheal neoplasms are unusual, although they occur slightly more frequently than benign primary tracheal neoplasms. Primary malignant neoplasms of the trachea often are due to squamous cell carcinoma, adenocarcinoma, or adenoid cystic carcinoma (the most common of the mixed salivary gland tumors or cylindromas). Carcinomas account for 60% to 90% of primary malignant tracheal neoplasms.[5] Less common are chondrosarcoma, fibrous sarcoma, carcinoid, and other rare mesenchymal tumors.

Tracheal squamous cell carcinoma represents just 0.1% of all primary malignancies. Malignant tumors above and below the trachea (laryngeal and bronchial) are 75 to 180 times more common. Tracheal squamous cell carcinomas arise most often in the caudal third of the trachea. These tumors are often sessile and eccentric, although 10% may be circumferential in contrast to benign tumors.

Chest radiographs are limited in the detection of tracheal tumors. CT, on the other hand, clearly shows the abnormal soft-tissue mass, usually arising from the posterior or lateral wall, as in this case. Also, up to 40% of tracheal squamous cell carcinomas may have mediastinal invasion, well seen on CT images. (Case courtesy of Nestor L. Müller, Vancouver, British Columbia.)

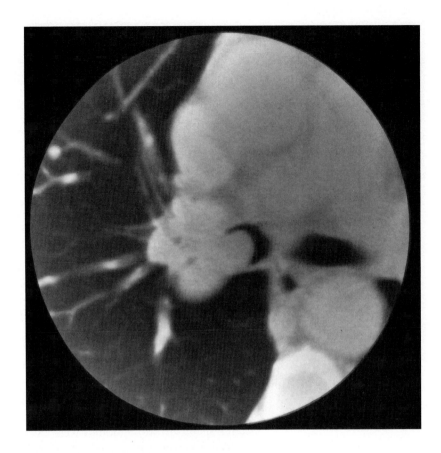

FIGURE 3-20

CT scan shows an 8 mm lesion arising from the lateral aspect of the right mainstem bronchus. It nearly occludes the airway. There was mild air trapping on expiratory views. Diagnosis was metastasis of uterine leiomyosarcoma.

Metastases to the trachea are unusual although more common than primary malignancies. They are seen in about 2% of patients dying from solid tumors and 5% of patients with multiple metastases.[6] The common primary tumors to metastasize to the trachea and bronchi are breast, colon, genitourinary (including testicular), melanoma, and now Kaposi's sarcoma. The radiographic and CT features are indistinguishable from those of central primary neoplasms.

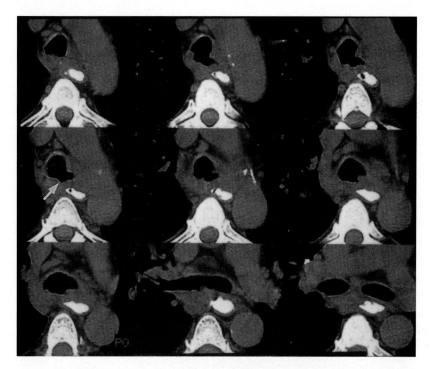

FIGURE 3-21
Serial CT scans through the midmediastinum show an infiltrative mass involving the distal trachea and mainstem bronchi. There is ulceration of the dorsal aspect of the distal trachea (*arrow*). Findings were caused by nonHodgkin's lymphoma.

Neoplasms of adjacent structures such as thyroid, lung, and, esophagus may invade the trachea and may actually be the most frequent neoplasms involving this structure.

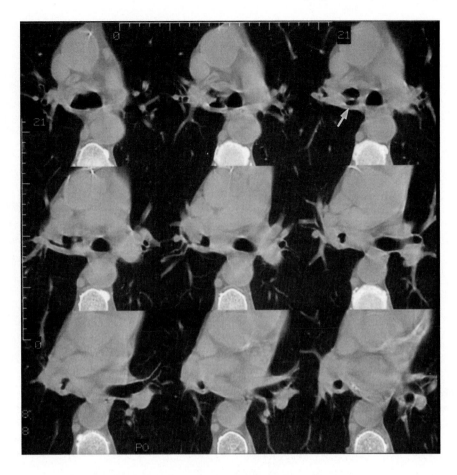

FIGURE 3-22

Serial CT scans through the hila show a soft-tissue infiltrative process around the right mainstem bronchus. There is fistulous communication to a cavity just dorsal to the right mainstem bronchus (*arrow*). There is infiltration around the bronchus intermedius, which is significantly narrowed. Findings were due to nonHodgkin's lymphoma.

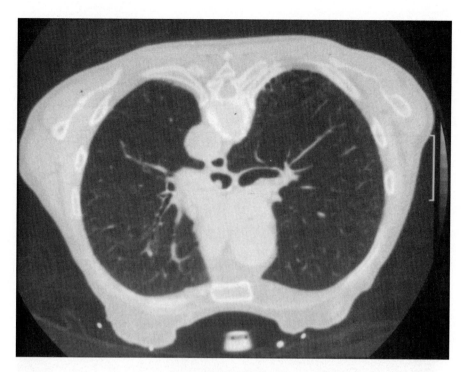

FIGURE 3-23

HRCT scan shows a 5 mm nodular lesion on the anterior wall of the left mainstem bronchus. This was observed on the CT monitor before the patient was released. Contiguous scans were obtained through this region after the patient was instructed to cough; the lesion resolved, and the diagnosis of adherent mucus was made.

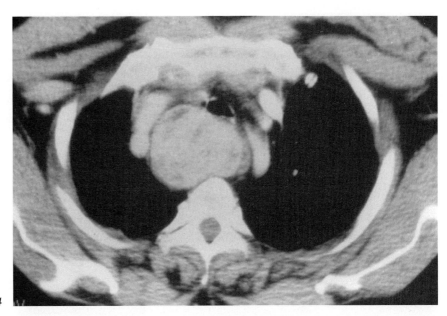

Figure 3-24

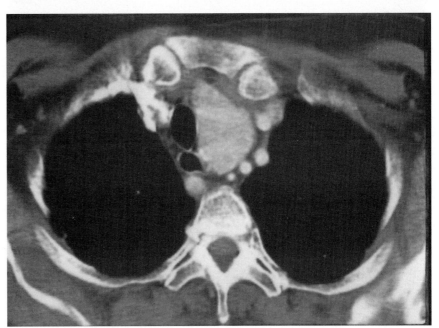

Figure 3-25

FIGURES 3-24 and 3-25

CT scans from two different patients with superior mediastinal masses both show a large hypervascular mass deviating the trachea and the great arterial vasculature. Cephalad images showed both masses to be connected to the thyroid. Findings are compatible with benign goiter, as was the surgical diagnosis. Thyroid goiters are often of relatively high attenuation before intravenous contrast material administration, given their natural iodine content. To make a diagnosis of goiter with CT, it must be shown that it is connected to the cervical thyroid gland. There are often punctate regions of calcification and low attenuation lesions within goiters.

Aberrant right subclavian artery aneurysm

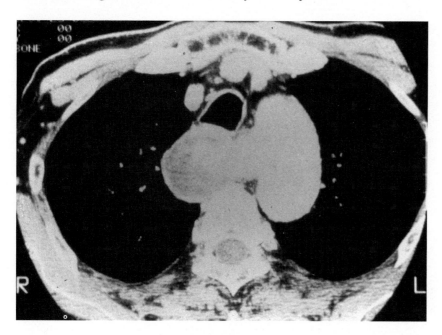

FIGURE 3-26

CT scan from a patient with an aberrant right subclavian artery aneurysm clearly shows the etiology of the deviated trachea. Benign enlargement or masses of adjacent structures such as this thyroid goiter or aberrant right subclavian artery aneurysm may displace the trachea.

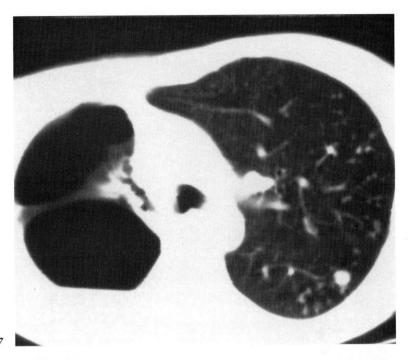

Figure 3-27

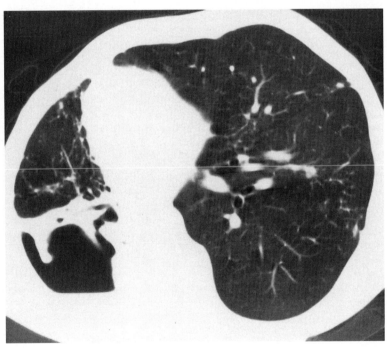

Figure 3-28

FIGURES 3-27 and 3-28

CT scans from these two patients show a dilated and tortuous airway leading into a large air-fluid collection in the pleural space: CT scan shows the bronchopleural fistula.

Tracheal diverticulum

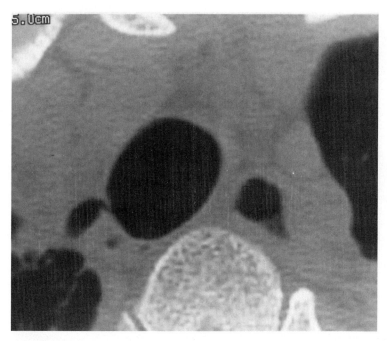

Figure 3-29

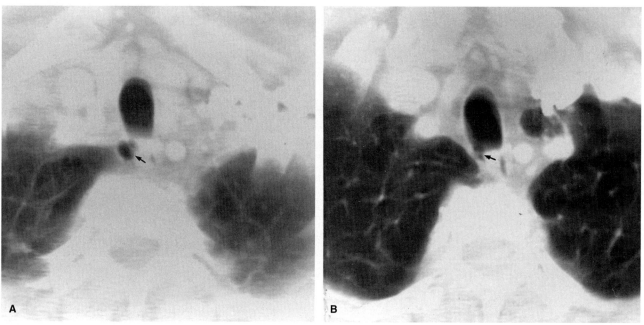

Figure 3-30

FIGURES 3-29 and 3-30

CT scans show two patients with tracheal diverticula extending posteriorly from the posterior membrane. These diverticula may extend cephalad or caudal, as illustrated in Figure 3-30 (*arrow*). These may occur with tracheobronchomegaly or may be incidental, as in these two patients.

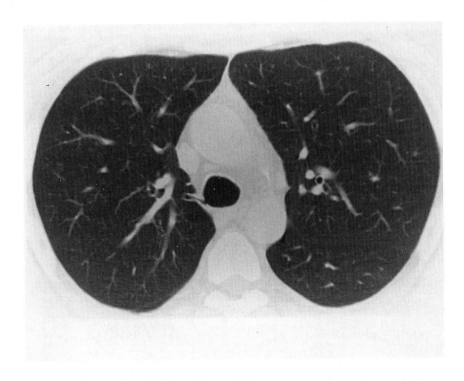

FIGURE 3-31

HRCT scan shows an anomalous bronchus to the right lung that arose just above the right mainstem bronchus. This may represent one of two conditions, often difficult to distinguish: a true supernumerary bronchus occurring in addition to the usual three upper lobe segmental bronchi, or an apical segmental bronchus displaced from the right upper lobe bronchus. A true supernumerary bronchus gives rise to a true tracheal lobe and is a normal finding in some mammals (e.g., pigs). In humans, such lobes are usually asymptomatic but can give rise to recurrent infections.

Tracheoesophageal fistula

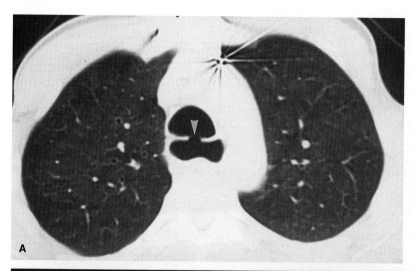

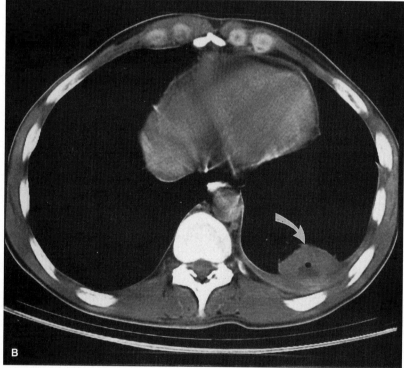

FIGURE 3-32

CT scan of the upper thorax shows a tracheoesophageal fistula (*arrowhead*). This tracheoesophageal fistula predisposed the patient to aspiration, which resulted in the left lower lobe lung abscess (*curved arrow*). Tracheoesophageal fistulas may result from endoscopy, surgery, lye ingestion, mediastinitis, radiation, neoplasm, or trauma.

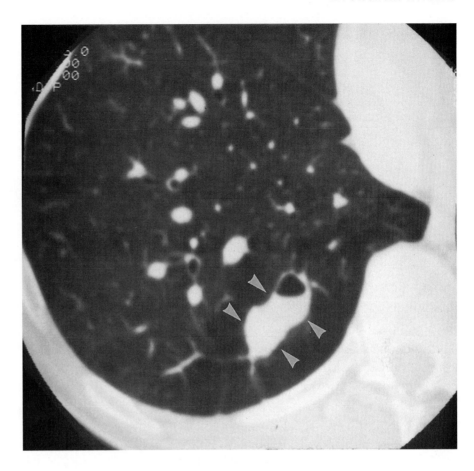

FIGURE 3-33

HRCT scan shows typical findings of bronchial atresia. There is a dilated bronchus that contains mucus and a small amount of air in the posterior basal segment of the right lower lobe (*arrowheads*). Note marked hyperlucency of lung surrounding the mucus-filled atretic bronchus.

Right middle lobe syndrome

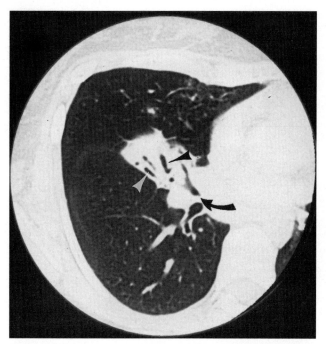

Figure 3-34

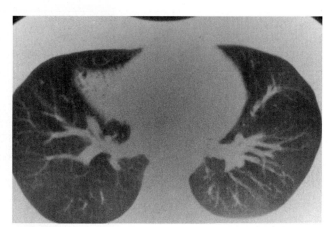

Figure 3-35

FIGURES 3-34 and 3-35

HRCT scans from two patients with right middle lobe syndrome show complete collapse of the middle lobe. There is ectasia of the visualized bronchi (*arrowheads*). In Figure 3-34, note that the middle lobe bronchus is patent (*curved arrow*). Both patients had a history of recurrent middle lobe infections. Bronchoscopy in each showed no obstructing lesion.

Right middle lobe syndrome is characterized by a spectrum of diseases, from recurrent atelectasis and pneumonia to bronchiectasis. In 60% of cases the cause is benign inflammation (e.g., tuberculous adenopathy or bronchostenosis). However, retained foreign body or tumor may also cause this syndrome and must be excluded. Some authors speculate that right middle lobe syndrome is related to relative isolation of the middle lobe, where lack of collateral ventilation impairs mucus clearance.

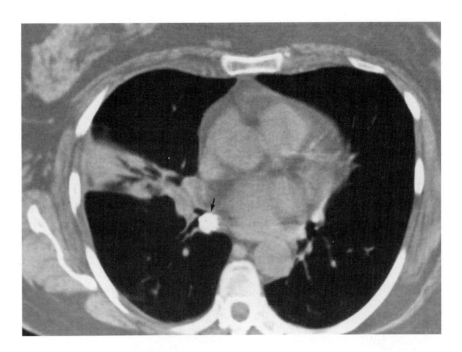

FIGURE 3-36

CT scan shows a large calcified lymph node eroding into the right main bronchus (*arrow*) with resultant parenchymal opacification (chronic) in the right middle lobe. In this patient, right middle lobe syndrome is secondary to prior histoplasmosis infection, now with erosive broncholith.

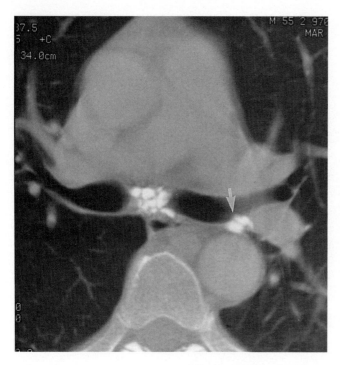

FIGURE 3-37

CT scan shows large calcified subcarinal and left hilar nodes secondary to histoplasmosis. In this case, the left hilar nodes were eroding through the airway (*arrow*), producing a broncholith that caused hemoptysis.

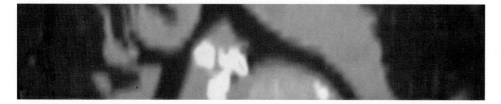

FIGURE 3-38

Coronal reconstruction of volumetric CT scans through the left mainstem bronchus shows a fistula from the left mainstem bronchus to calcified subcarinal nodes. This patient presented with a history of lithoptysis, and this CT examination confirmed the presumed diagnosis of broncholithiasis.

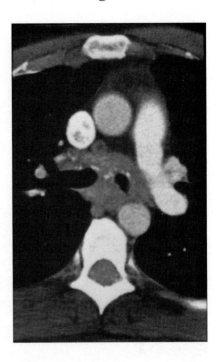

FIGURE 3-39

Contrast-enhanced CT scan through the mainstem bronchi shows an infiltrative mass surrounding these airways. There is mild narrowing of the left mainstem bronchus. A small amount of calcification within this process is also present. These findings were shown to be produced by fibrosing mediastinitis secondary to histoplasmosis. Differential diagnostic considerations include lymphoma.

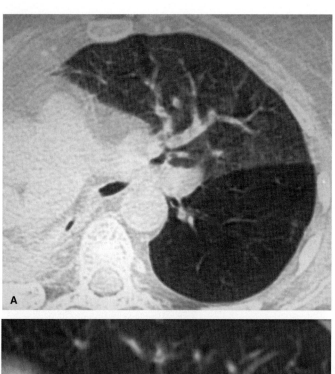

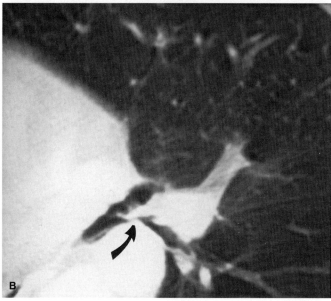

FIGURE 3-40

This patient developed new onset of dyspnea after right pneumonectomy. The chest radiograph showed only normal postoperative findings of pneumonectomy. Expiratory CT scan (A) shows air trapping in the left lower lobe. The left upper lobe deflated normally. Note also the marked relative oligemia of the left lower lobe compared to the upper lobe. HRCT scan (B) shows marked narrowing of the left lower lobe bronchus, where it is tethered over the descending aorta. Findings are compatible with postpneumonectomy syndrome and are secondary to stretching and extrinsic pressure on the lower lobe bronchus. Surgery to reposition the mediastinum more centrally with prosthetic filling of the right thorax was helpful in alleviating the left lower lobe bronchial obstruction in this patient.

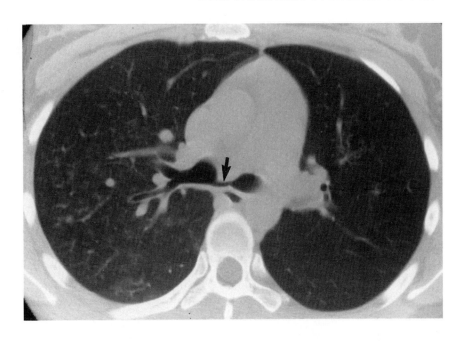

FIGURE 3-41

CT scan shows the results of a traumatic rupture of the left main bronchus many years before, now with severe stenosis of the bronchus (*arrow*). Note the resulting air trapping in the left lower lobe. Ventilation-perfusion study revealed 1% of total ventilation and 12% of total perfusion in the left lung. Incidental bronchoalveolar lavage fluid in the right lung produced patchy ground-glass opacification.

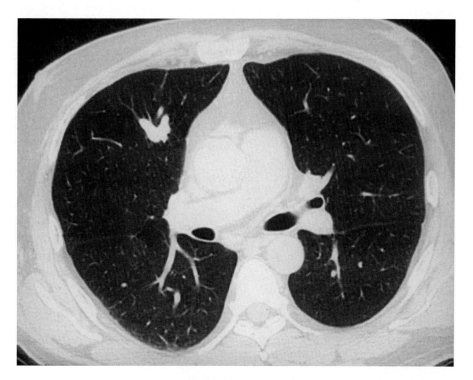

FIGURE 3-42

HRCT scan shows a branched tubular structure in the anterior segment of the right upper lobe. This finding is compatible with a mucoid impaction (see Figs. 7-33, 7-43); however, endobronchial metastasis can have an identical appearance. This patient had a renal cell carcinoma, and this focal lung lesion was shown to be an endobronchial metastasis.

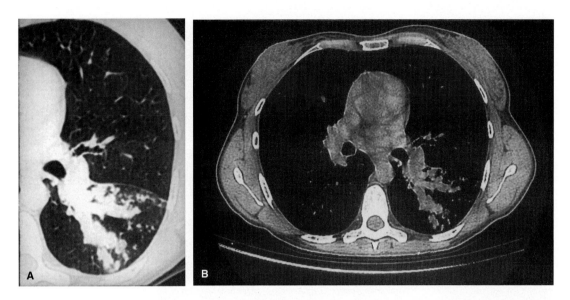

FIGURE 3-43

An inverted, V-shaped, branching tubular structure in the superior segment of the left lower lobe is characteristic of mucoid impaction on this HRCT scan (lung and soft-tissue windows) of an asthmatic patient with allergic bronchopulmonary aspergillosis. Central bronchiectasis and mucoid impaction are common findings in patients with this disease.

Atypical carcinoid tumor with mucoid impaction

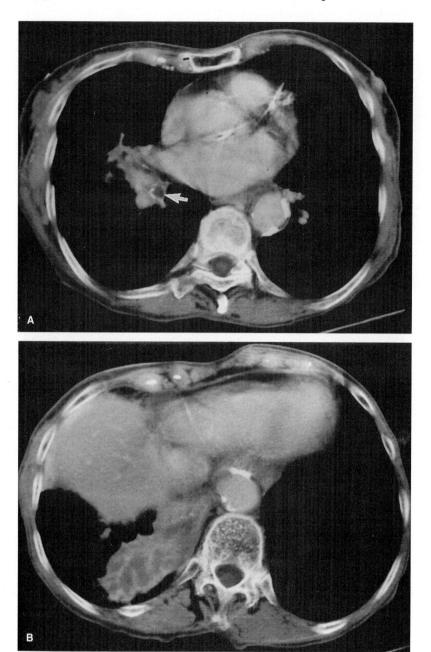

FIGURE 3-44

CT scan from a patient with an atypical carcinoid tumor in the bronchus intermedius (*arrow*) shows mucoid impaction. Note the relatively low attenuation of mucus in the branching bronchi compared with the surrounding enhancing lung parenchyma.

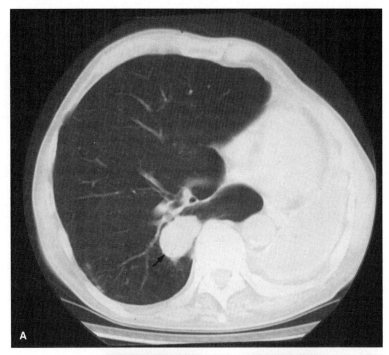

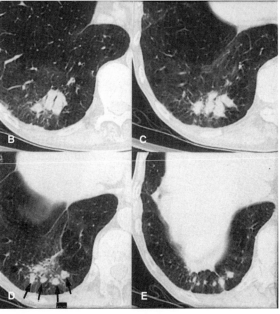

FIGURE 3-45

Serial contiguous HRCT scans show a 3 cm mass in the posterior basal segment of the right lower lobe (*arrow*). Note branched tubular structures inferior to this mass. Findings were caused by an obstructing squamous cell carcinoma with distal mucoid impaction in subsegmental bronchi (*arrows*); parenchymal aeration was maintained by collateral air drift. Mucoid impaction may be caused by an obstructing lesion such as endobronchial tumor, bronchostenosis, or broncholithiasis. Other diagnostic considerations include asthma, allergic bronchopulmonary aspergillosis, dysmotile cilia syndrome, and postoperative pulmonary status.

REFERENCES

1. Dunne MG, Reiner B. CT features of tracheobronchomegaly. J Comput Assist Tomogr 1988; 12:388–391

2. Meyer E, Dinkel E, Nilles A. Tracheobronchomegaly: Clinical aspects and radiological features. Eur J Radiol 1990; 10:126–129

3. Greene R, Lechner GL. "Saber-sheath" trachea: A clinical and functional study of marked coronal narrowing of the intrathoracic trachea. Radiology 1975; 115:265–268

4. Im JG, Chung JW, Han SK, Han MC, Kim CW. CT manifestations of tracheobronchial involvement in relapsing polychondritis. J Comput Assist Tomogr 1988; 12:792–793

5. Grillo HC, Mathisen DJ, Wain JC. Management of tumors of the trachea. Oncology (Williston Park) 1992; 6:61–67

6. Piacenza G, Mantellini E, Cremonte LG, Salio M. Isolated endobronchial metastases. Minerva Med 1986; 77:1793–1794

High-Resolution CT of the Chest: Comprehensive Atlas
by Eric J. Stern and Stephen J. Swensen,
Lippincott–Raven Publishers, Philadelphia © 1996.

Bronchiectasis

4

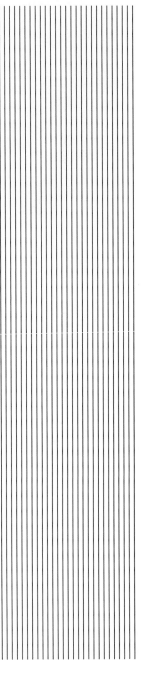

Bronchiectasis

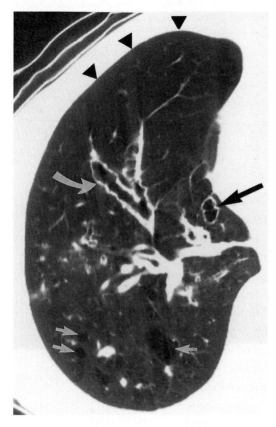

FIGURE 4-1

HRCT scan shows the difference between emphysematous spaces (*small white arrows*), bronchiectatic airways in cross-sectional (*black arrow*) and longitudinal planes (*curved white arrow*), and air trapping (*arrowheads*).

Bronchiectasis is a chronic, usually inflammatory, often suppurative condition that leads to irreversibly dilated airways. Depending upon severity, the HRCT signs of bronchiectasis include bronchial wall thickening caused by peribronchial inflammation and fibrosis, dilated bronchi in the periphery of the lung, air-fluid levels in distended bronchi, and a linear array or cluster of cystlike spaces. Distended bronchi are easily distinguished from bullae, which generally have no definable wall thickness and no accompanying vessels.

Although bronchiectasis has been classically categorized into cylindrical, varicose, and saccular (cystic) types, the spectrum of disease may prevent neat classification in patients with varying degrees of severity in different regions of the lung. Because these categories have little clinical use, they are used infrequently in current practice.

Cylindrical bronchiectasis is the least severe form. Varicose bronchiectasis produces alternating dilatation and constriction, yielding a beaded, varicoid appearance. Saccular and cystic bronchiectasis are the most severe forms; in them, the airways are markedly dilated. In patients with bronchiectasis, there is occasionally concomitant severe parenchymal destruction and obliteration of the distal airways (obliterative bronchiolitis) (*arrowheads*).

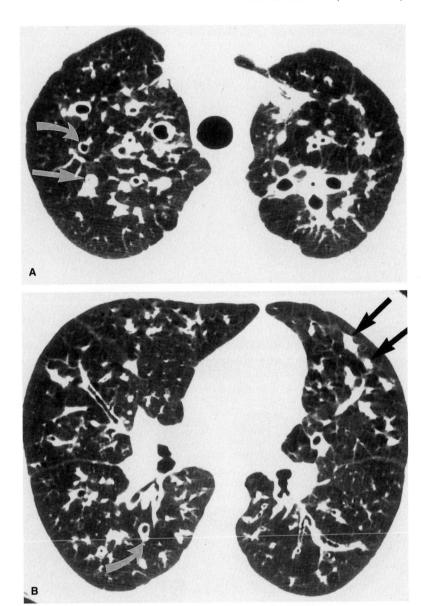

FIGURE 4-2

HRCT scans show multiple dilated bronchiectatic airways that form the classic signet-ring sign with their accompanying pulmonary artery (*curved arrow*). Also note the mucoid impaction (*straight arrows*).

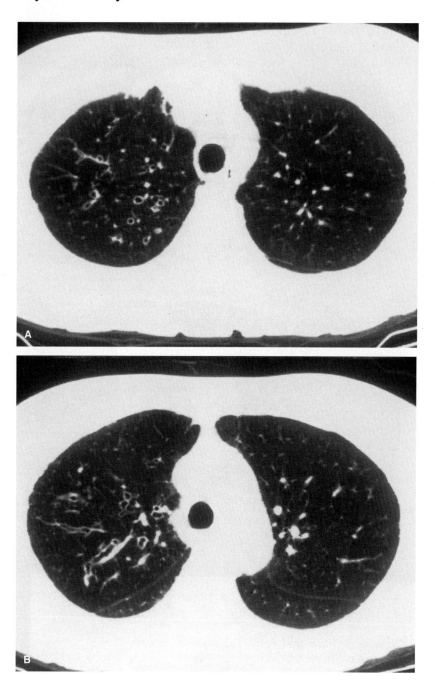

FIGURE 4-3

Bronchiectasis is not always diffuse or symmetric. HRCT scans show cylindrical bronchiectasis in the right upper lobe in contrast with the normal airways of the left upper lobe.

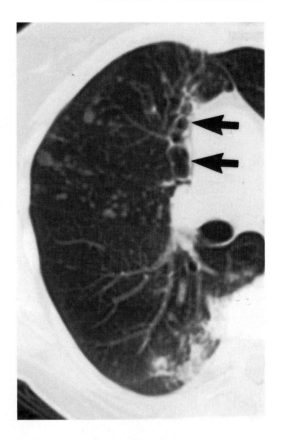

FIGURE 4-4

CT scan shows findings of varicose bronchiectasis. Note "string of pearl" or varicose appearance of abnormally tapering and dilated bronchus (*arrows*). There are four classifications of bronchiectasis in increasing order of severity: cylindical, varicose, saccular, and cystic. The nodules in this case are caused by *Mycobacterium avium-intracellulare.*

Saccular bronchiectasis

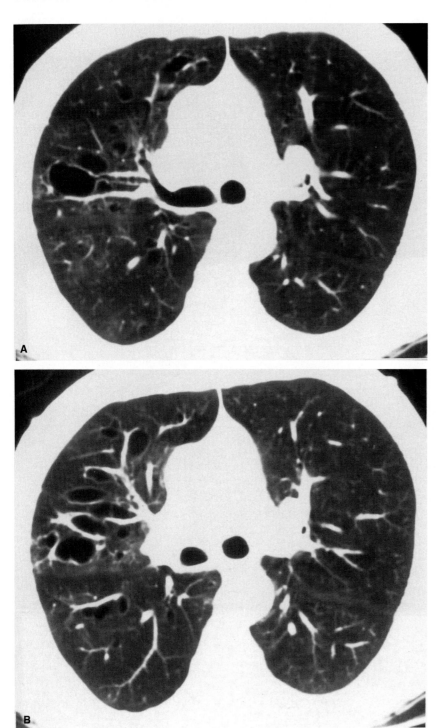

FIGURE 4-5

HRCT scans show marked dilatation and airway wall thickening of multiple small to moderate sized airways in the right middle and lower lobes. Although the central bronchi are normal, the presence of marked dilatation and thickened walls in small and moderate airways indicates saccular bronchiectasis peripherally.

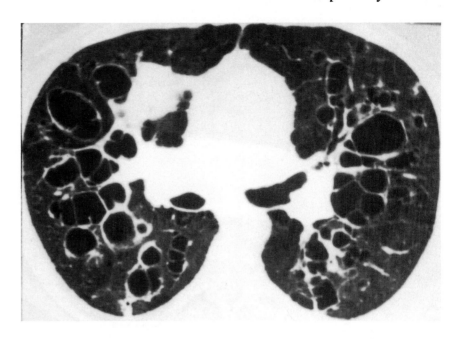

FIGURE 4-6

HRCT scan from this patient with Williams-Campbell syndrome shows extensive changes of saccular bronchiectasis. Williams-Campbell syndrome is congenital bronchomalacia owing to the absence of annular cartilage distal to the first division of the bronchi. There is characteristically advanced bronchiectasis. (Case courtesy of Steve L. Primack, University of Oregon, Portland.)

Cystic bronchiectasis

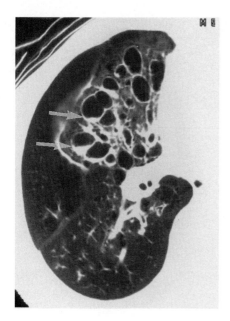

FIGURE 4-7

HRCT scan shows multiple rounded lucencies with discrete walls representing severe cystic bronchiectasis almost entirely replacing the middle lobe. Note air-fluid levels in some bronchi (*arrows*).

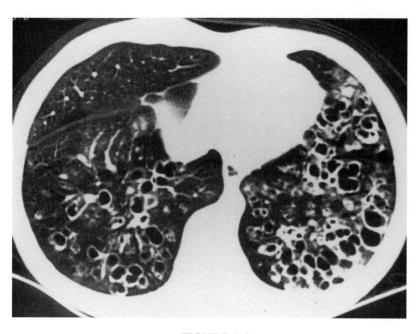

FIGURE 4-8

HRCT scan in this patient who suffered an episode of pneumonia in childhood shows extensive cystic bronchiectasis. When it is severe, bronchiectasis can appear very similar to cystic lung diseases (see Chapter 6). Cystic bronchiectatic airways can usually be followed over serial CT slices and shown to be contiguous with one another; the cross-section of a tubular structure appears round and cystic.

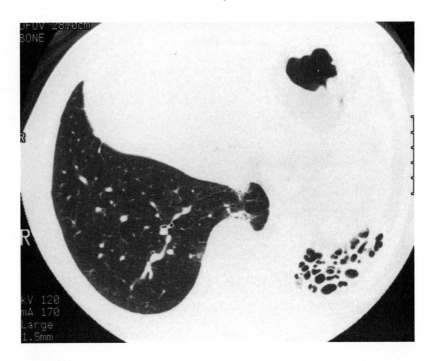

FIGURE 4-9

HRCT scan shows unilateral bronchiectasis in this patient whose left lung parenchyma was destroyed by tuberculosis. Bronchiectasis of this severity does not necessarily imply remote or longstanding infection. Postprimary tuberculosis may cause this amount of lung destruction in as little as 6 to 12 months.

Bronchiectasis

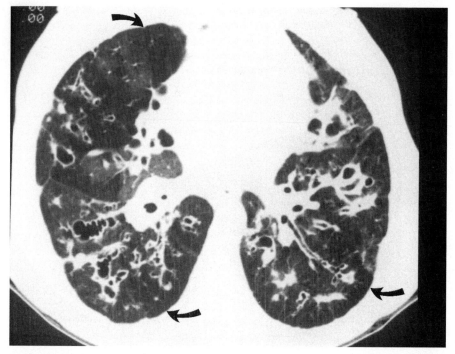

Figure 4-10

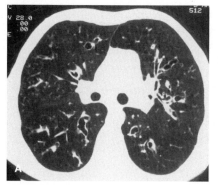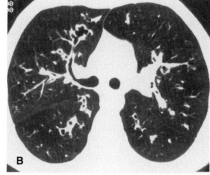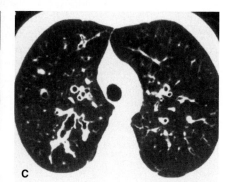

Figure 4-11

FIGURES 4-10 and 4-11

HRCT scans show multiple irregularly shaped bronchiectatic airways in two patients with cystic fibrosis. Bronchiectatic airways can attain different, often bizarre shapes even in the same patient, reflecting an often chronic and ongoing inflammatory airways disease. Note mosaic pattern of lung parenchymal attenuation. Hyperlucent regions are due to air trapping (*arrows*) in this case.

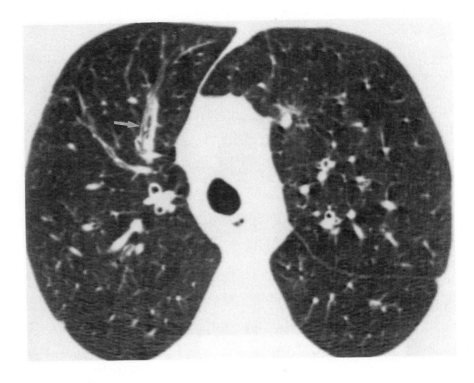

FIGURE 4-12

HRCT scan shows mild central bronchial wall thickening (*arrow*) and dilatation (bronchiectasis) in a patient with asthma. This combination of clinical and CT findings suggests allergic bronchopulmonary aspergillosis, a destructive inflammatory disease of the airways. Patients with this disease usually have an immediate cutaneous reaction to a challenge with *Aspergillus fumigatus*.[1]

Bronchiectasis secondary to chronic granulomatous disease of childhood

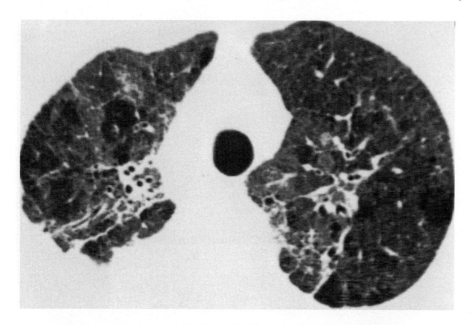

FIGURE 4-13

HRCT scan shows bilateral parenchymal scarring, architectural distortion, and bronchiectasis, worse in the right lung. These chronic inflammatory changes are caused by chronic granulomatous disease of childhood. This rare, genetically heterogeneous, inherited disorder is characterized by repeated infections of the skin, lymph nodes, and viscera. The lung is the most common site of infection, and lung disease is the primary cause of death in more than 50% of affected children.

In chronic granulomatous disease of childhood, the ability of phagocytes to kill ingested microorganisms is severely hampered by a deficiency of nicotinamide-adenine dinucleotide phosphate oxidase. Affected tissues respond with a granulomatous reaction. The most common infecting agents are staphylococci, gram-negative organisms, *Candida* and *Aspergillus*.

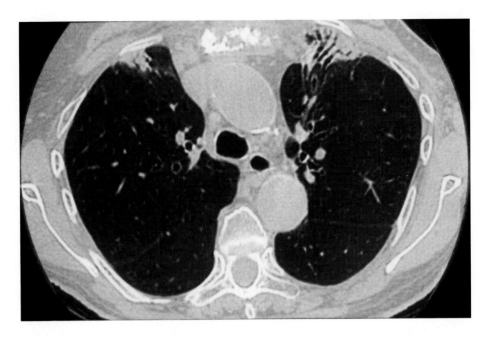

FIGURE 4-14

HRCT scan shows a fibrotic infiltrative process in the anterior aspects of the lungs with consequent traction bronchiectasis. This patient had metastatic spread of breast carcinoma to the sternum, for which she received radiation therapy. Note that the distribution of fibrosis does not conform to any normal segmental or lobar lung anatomy; rather, it reflects the radiation port, often presenting in a geometric, nonanatomic pattern.

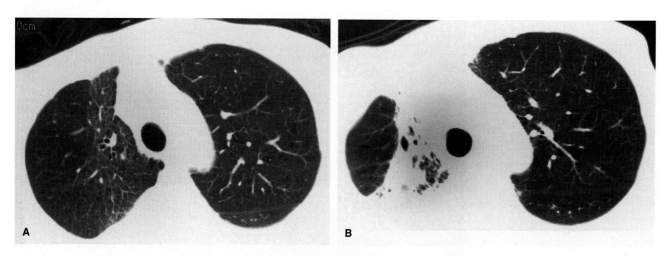

FIGURE 4-15

HRCT scan (A) shows characteristic findings of radiation pneumonitis. Note the straight, nonanatomic border that marginates the area of abnormality in the medial right lung. This corresponds to the radiation port.

HRCT scan performed 15 months later (B) shows marked volume loss in the right hemithorax with architectural distortion, including cystic changes and traction bronchiectasis in the irradiated segment. The nonanatomic border of the abnormal area, reflecting the previous radiation port, persists.

Findings of radiation pneumonitis usually are apparent on CT within 16 weeks of radiotherapy; however, they can be detected as early as 4 weeks after completion of radiotherapy.[2] There can be progression of injury for several months, but by 6 to 9 months after radiation therapy has been completed, the injury stabilizes, and healing with subsequent scarring begins.

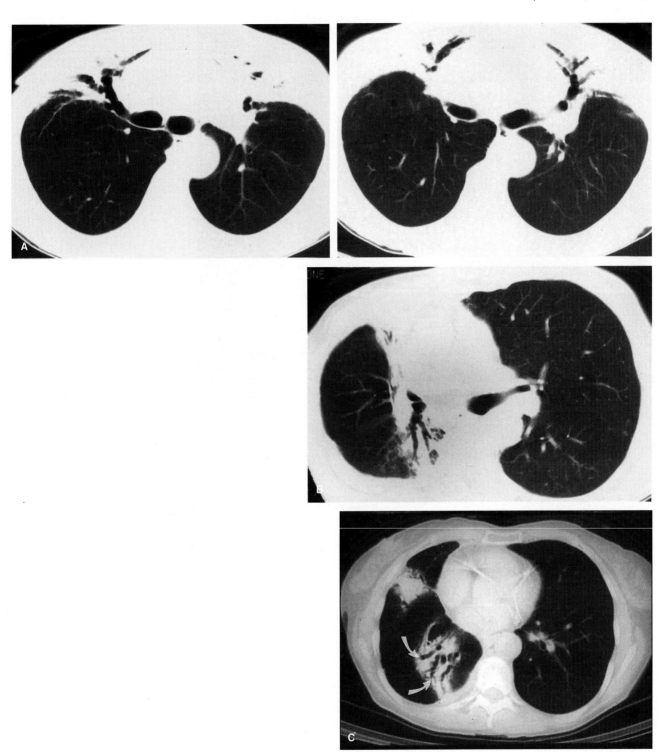

FIGURE 4-16

HRCT scan appearances of bronchiectasis secondary to radiation fibrosis in three patients. The bronchiectasis (*arrows*) that develops is caused by cicatrization and consequent traction, reflecting the intense fibrotic nature of late-stage radiation pneumonitis. It is not caused by intrinsic disease of the airways.[3]

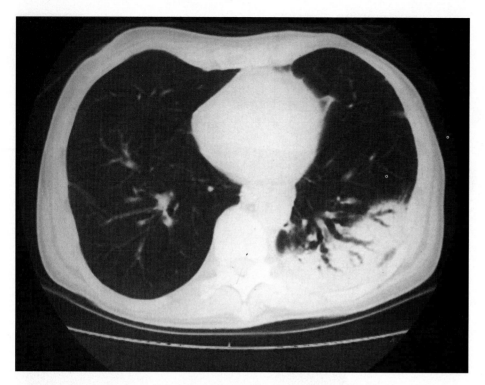

FIGURE 4-17

CT scan of a patient with aspiration pneumonia in the left lower lobe shows bronchial dilatation within the region of disease. Subsequent HRCT examination showed that the airways had returned to normal caliber.

In pneumonia or atelectasis, the airways may dilate transiently. This "reversible bronchiectasis" is probably related to alterations in airway compliance and parenchymal stresses. Because reversible bronchiectasis may be present in patients who have recently had a suppurative pneumonia, consider delaying a HRCT examination for the diagnosis of bronchiectasis at least 3 to 6 months after the resolution of the infection in order to avoid a false diagnosis of bronchiectasis.

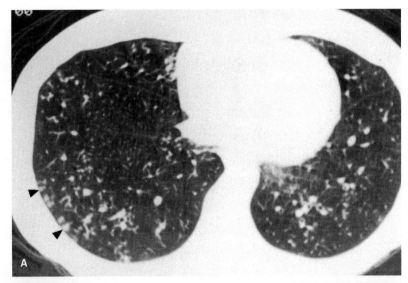

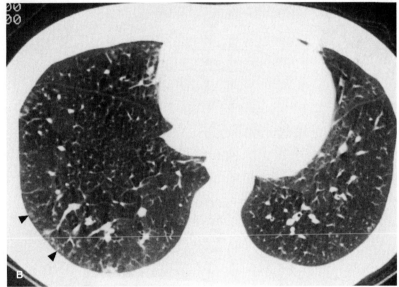

FIGURE 4-18

HRCT scan shows (A) multiple, peripheral, irregular nodules in both lower lobes (*arrowheads*). In this patient with a diagnosis of yellow nail syndrome, these nodules represent mildly dilated, mucus-filled bronchioles.

Yellow nail syndrome is an unusual lymphangitic disorder that may be due to congenital hypoplasia of the lymphatics. It is characterized by a classic triad of physical findings: yellow nail discoloration, lymphedema, and pleural effusion that may be chylous or exudative. Bronchiectasis with bronchial wall thickening, bronchial dilatation, and mucus plugging is an associated pulmonary feature.

After medical treatment of this patient, mucus plugging partially resolved; HRCT scan (B) showed a decrease in the size and number of the peripherally mucus-plugged small bronchi (*arrowheads*).[4]

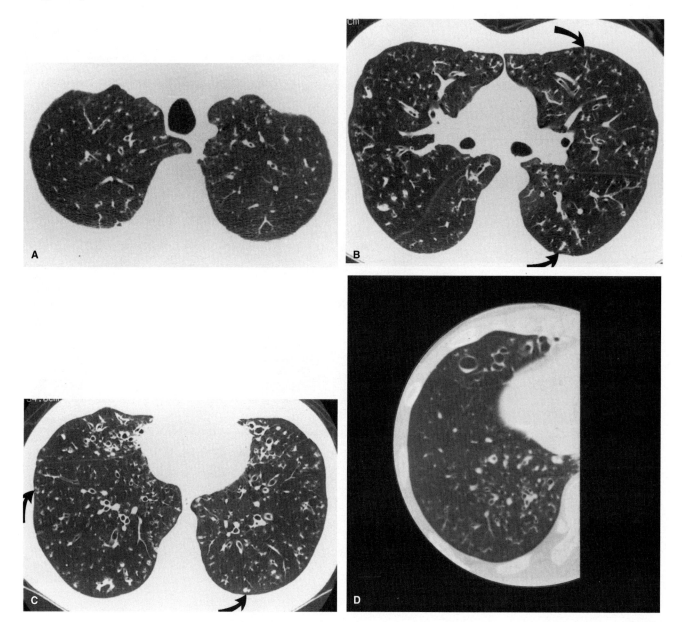

FIGURE 4-19

HRCT scans from two patients with diffuse panbronchiolitis (A–C and D) show diffuse ectasia of bronchi and bronchioles and numerous small nodular and linear opacities, centrally located in secondary pulmonary lobules. The small nodular and linear opacities represent dilated bronchioles filled with intrabronchial fibrosis or secretion (*arrows*).[5] In (D), there are several dilated airways with air-fluid levels. This is a chronic idiopathic disease of bronchi and bronchioles, primarily affecting those of Asian origin, characterized by chronic air flow limitation and diffuse airway inflammation.

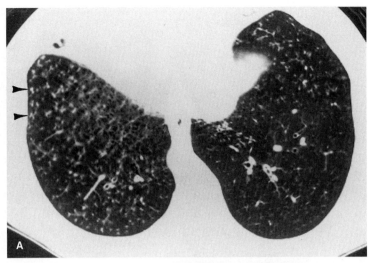

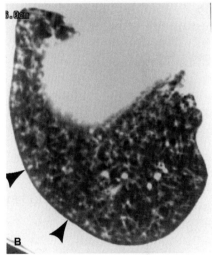

FIGURE 4-20

HRCT scans show numerous dilated and mucus-filled bronchioles with thick walls that have the appearance of small, ill-defined nodules (*arrowheads*). This patient had situs inversus and was diagnosed as having Kartagener's syndrome. The HRCT presence of bronchiectasis and bronchiolectasis supports this diagnosis.

Dysmotile cilia syndromes result in chronic infection of the airways and sinuses, infertility in males, and a high incidence of abnormal thoracic, cardiac, and/or abdominal situs. When situs inversus totalis is present, the syndrome is classified as Kartagener's. In patients with abnormal cilia, bronchial clearance of mucus is impaired, and chronic infection with bronchiectasis results. Dilatation of central or segmental bronchi may be present, or those airways may appear normal with only bronchiolectasis evident. Unlike panbronchiolitis, which is diffusely distributed, bronchiectasis and bronchiolectasis in dysmotile cilia syndromes are usually confined to the lung bases, probably because of the exacerbation of the impaired mucus clearance by gravity.

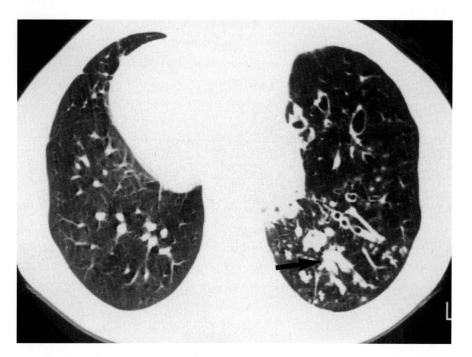

FIGURE 4-21

HRCT scan shows bronchiectasis and dextrocardia in this patient with Kartagener's syndrome. Note the mucoid impaction (*arrow*). Asymmetry of the bronchiectasis does not exclude this diagnosis. Figures 4-20 and 4-21 show the spectrum of bronchiectasis that occurs in Kartagener's syndrome.

REFERENCES

1.   Neeld DA, Goodman LR, Gurney JW, Greenberger PA, Fink JN. Computerized tomography in the evaluation of allergic bronchopulmonary aspergillosis. Am Rev Respir Dis 1990; 142:1200–1205

2.   Ikezoe J, Takashima S, Morimoto S, et al. CT appearance of acute radiation-induced injury in the lung. AJR 1988; 150:765–770

3.   Libshitz HI, Shuman LS. Radiation-induced pulmonary change: CT findings. J Comput Assist Tomogr 1984; 8:15–19

4.   Wiggins J, Strickland B, Chung KF. Detection of bronchiectasis by high-resolution computed tomography in the yellow nail syndrome. Clin Radiol 1991; 43:377–379

5.   Nishimura K, Kitaichi M, Izumi T, Itoh H. Diffuse panbronchiolitis: Correlation of high-resolution CT and pathologic findings. Radiology 1992; 184:779–785

High-Resolution CT of the Chest: Comprehensive Atlas
by Eric J. Stern and Stephen J. Swensen,
Lippincott–Raven Publishers, Philadelphia © 1996.

Small Airways Diseases

5

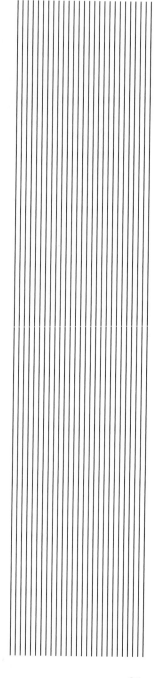

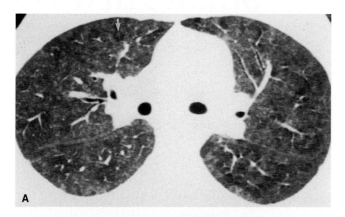

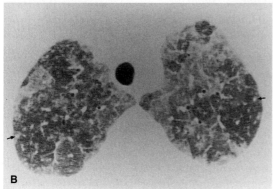
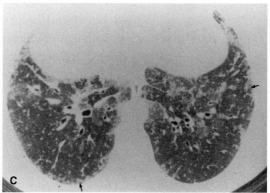

FIGURE 5-1

HRCT scans from these two patients—(A) and (B, C)—show a mosaic of ground-glass opacification and small, hazy, ill-defined nodular opacities (*arrows*) centered around peripheral bronchovascular bundles—small airways—consistent with hypersensitivity pneumonitis. Depending on chronicity, the ground-glass opacity can be caused by noncaseating granulomas, filling of the air spaces with macrophages, interstitial pneumonitis, and bronchiolitis.[1]

Hypersensitivity pneumonitis (also called extrinsic allergic alveolitis) occurs in response to the inhalation of organic particles in the home or workplace. It may be acute, subacute, or chronic. This immunologically mediated disease is often difficult to distinguish clinically and physiologically from other idiopathic diffuse lung diseases. The diagnosis is usually based on a constellation of findings that include antigen exposure, characteristic signs and symptoms, abnormal physical examination, and physiologic and radiographic evaluation.

In patients with hypersensitivity pneumonitis, the chest radiograph commonly appears normal. HRCT is more sensitive than a chest radiograph for the detection of this disease.[2]

Two widely recognized types of hypersensitivity pneumonitis are farmer's lung and bird-fancier's lung. Numerous other antigenic substances have also been recognized.[3]

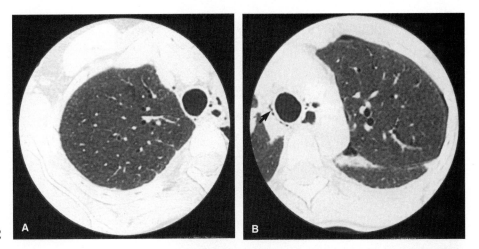

Figure 5-2

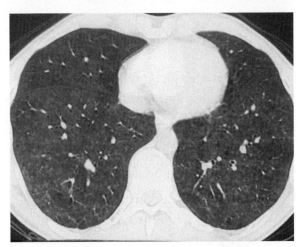

Figure 5-3

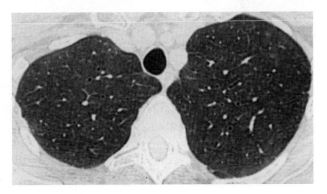

Figure 5-4

FIGURES 5-2, 5-3, and 5-4

HRCT scans from three patients with subacute bird-fancier's lung show common characteristic findings: diffuse, poorly circumscribed, small nodular opacities that involve peribronchiolar tissues (centrilobular). Also noted are regions of poorly circumscribed ground-glass opacity that correlate histologically with interstitial pneumonitis, cellular bronchiolitis, and small, noncaseating granulomas.[1] Air trapping may also be present in some patients.[4] Note the pneumothorax and pneumomediastinum (*arrow*) in Figure 5–2B: these were presumed to have been caused by paroxysmal coughing.

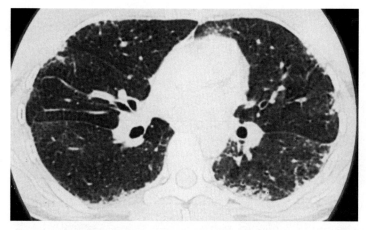

Figure 5-5

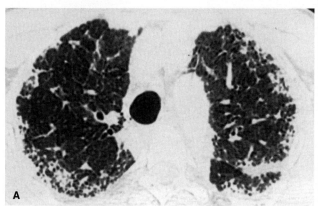

Figure 5-6

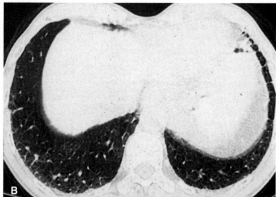

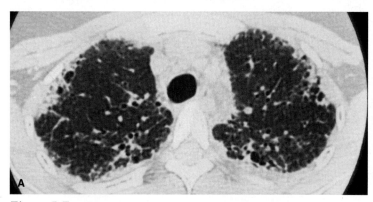

Figure 5-7

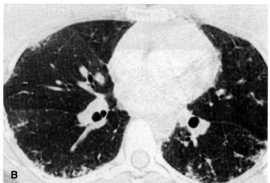

FIGURES 5-5, 5-6, and 5-7

HRCT scans from three patients shown to have bird-fancier's disease causing chronic hypersensitivity pneumonitis, whose symptoms persisted for at least 12 months. A peripheral fibrotic process can be seen affecting the middle and upper lungs predominantly, with relative sparing of the apices and bases. However, other patients with chronic hypersensitivity pneumonitis may show diffuse disease without zonal predominance. This nonbasal distribution of fibrosis allows distinction of chronic hypersensitivity pneumonitis from other causes and types of fibrosis, such as idiopathic pulmonary fibrosis (see Figs. 8-1 through 8-10).[5]

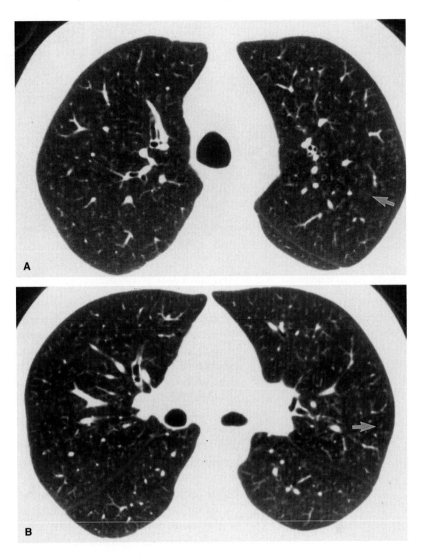

FIGURE 5-8

HRCT scans in this patient with graft-versus-host disease show diffuse small, ill-defined nodules (*arrows*). These parenchymal micronodules, arising in peribronchiolar locations, are related to inflammation and dilatation of the bronchioles (bronchiolitis/bronchiolectasis) and associated peribronchiolar fibrosis. The nodular opacities are very similar in appearance to those produced by the respiratory bronchiolitis seen in cigarette smokers (see Fig. 7-30 through 7-33).

Patients with acute and chronic graft-versus-host disease following allogeneic bone marrow transplantation rarely manifest small airway damage as one of the facets of graft-versus-host disease. The spectrum of small airway pathology can vary from early bronchiolar wall damage to bronchiolitis obliterans. The diagnosis is made in the proper clinical setting, in the absence of other identifiable pathogens of bronchiolitis obliterans.[6]

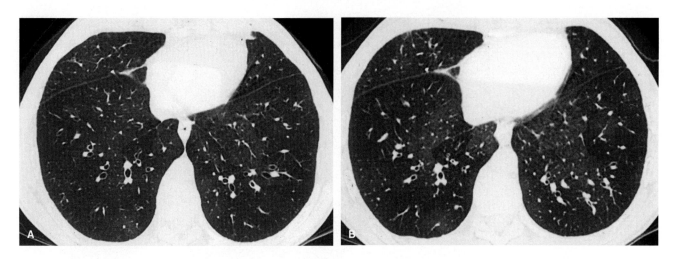

FIGURE 5-9

HRCT scan (A) obtained at full suspended inspiration. There is a slight inhomogeneity in the attenuation of the lung parenchyma. This represents air trapping, which, when severe, can be visible on inspiratory CT scans. HRCT scan (B) obtained at suspended full expiration at the same anatomic level as (A) shows multiple focal lucencies. These lucencies correspond to multiple secondary lobules and represent extensive air trapping in them. This indicates severe obstructive disease of the small airways in this patient with obliterative bronchiolitis.

Obliterative bronchiolitis (bronchiolitis obliterans) is a disease that can lead to progressive chronic respiratory failure. The underlying causes and predisposing factors for the development of obliterative bronchiolitis are many and include penicillamine therapy, previous infection (especially with measles or adenoviruses), graft-versus-host disease, collagen vascular disease (such as rheumatoid arthritis and polymyositis), and chronic lung allograft rejection.

In obliterative bronchiolitis, noncartilaginous bronchioles are occluded by granulation tissue and destroyed. The characteristic combination of clinical and physiologic features and evidence of air trapping at suspended full expiration HRCT often suggest the diagnosis of obliterative bronchiolitis.

Obliterative bronchiolitis: Air trapping evident on inspiratory and expiratory images

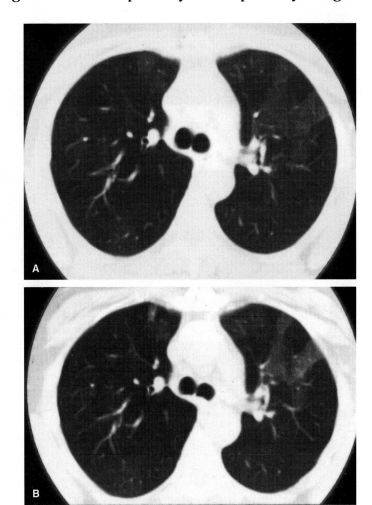

FIGURE 5-10

Inspiration (A) and expiration (B) CT scans show characteristic findings of obliterative bronchiolitis. Extensive air trapping is detectable on both the inspiratory and expiratory examinations. Note that with expiration the lucent regions of lung remain lucent, whereas the normal unobstructed lung becomes more opaque. These findings are nonspecific but indicate obstruction at the bronchiolar level.[7]

Air trapping that occurs as a result of disease of the small airways may be classified as fixed or reactive. In fixed obstruction, there is narrowing or occlusion of the small airways; this is a common feature in diffuse panbronchiolitis and obliterative bronchiolitis. Reactive disease is an intermittent process in which the small airways narrow, producing a temporary increase in resistance to air flow. Asthma and other forms of bronchospasm, including that which occurs in conjunction with chronic obstructive pulmonary disease, are classified as reactive airways disease.

Obliterative bronchiolitis: Mosaic pattern and hypoxic vasoconstriction

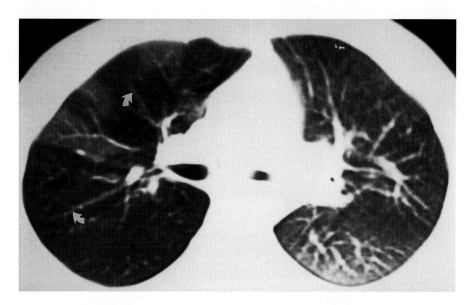

FIGURE 5-11

HRCT scan shows a mosaic pattern of lung attenuation. Again, it is the lucent regions of the right lung that are abnormal, whereas the more opaque regions in it as well as the entire left lung are normal. Note the reduced size of the vessels in the right lung (*arrows*) representing hypoxic vasoconstriction owing to decreased ventilation.

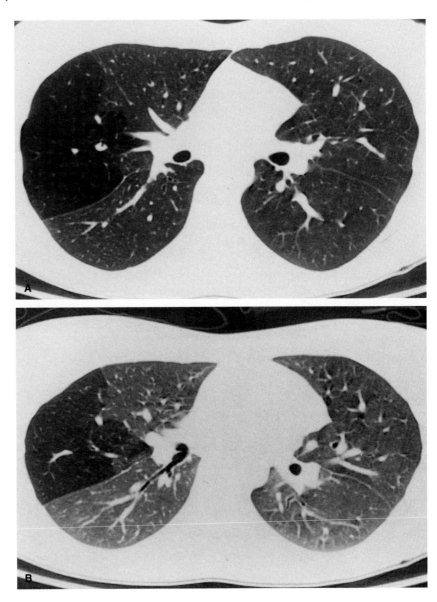

FIGURE 5-12

HRCT scans at inspiration (A) and expiration (B) show a markedly hyperlucent oligemic and expanded lateral segment of the middle lobe. This segment remains hyperlucent on the expiratory image. The rest of the right lung and left lung deflate normally. These findings indicate obstruction of the lateral segmental bronchus of the middle lobe. This finding is compatible with the clinical diagnosis of Swyer-James syndrome consequent to obliterative bronchiolitis. Swyer-James syndrome is usually caused by a childhood viral infection that results in bronchiectasis and obliterative bronchiolitis. On the chest radiograph, patients with Swyer-James syndrome classically have unilateral hyperlucent lung. On CT, the findings are often bilateral but asymmetric.[8] (Case courtesy of J. Takasugi, Seattle, Washington.)

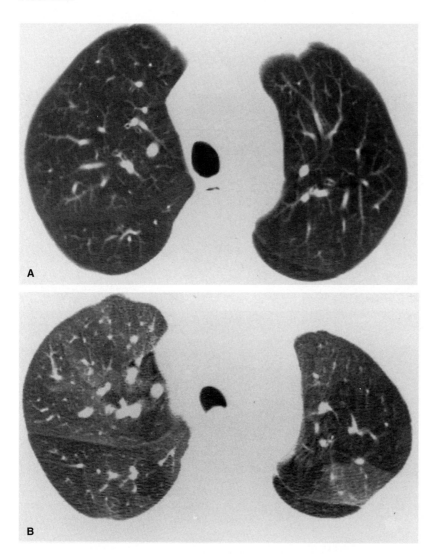

FIGURE 5-13

HRCT scan in this patient with asthma obtained at suspended full inspiration (A) produced images without detectable disease. However, repeat HRCT scan at suspended full expiration (B) shows patchy, inhomogeneous lung attenuation consistent with air trapping, a nonspecific but key finding that reflects obstruction to air flow in small bronchi and bronchioli.

In patients with small airways diseases, HRCT scans obtained at suspended full inspiration may be entirely normal, as in this patient. Expiratory CT scanning can play an important role in the diagnostic work-up of patients with small airways diseases. It is very sensitive in detecting subtle air trapping, in many cases more sensitive than spirometry;[9] the detection of air trapping can provide clues to an otherwise unsuspected or underappreciated small airways disease. Expiratory CT scanning provides both anatomic and physiologic information that is complementary to both conventional suspended full-inspiration CT and pulmonary function testing. Depending on the clinical scenario, the extent and distribution of air trapping are useful in indicating or directing further diagnostic work-up, such as transbronchial, thoracoscopic, or open lung biopsy.

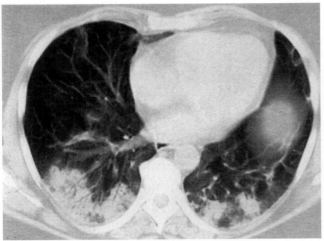 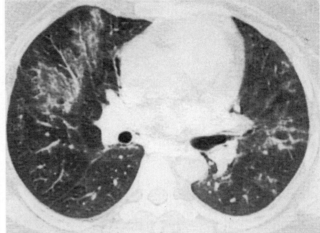

Figure 5-14   *Figure 5-15*

FIGURES 5-14 and 5-15

HRCT scans from these two patients with bronchiolitis obliterans–organizing pneumonia (BOOP) show multiple peripheral, nonspecific areas of consolidated lung
parenchyma. Although some of these areas are well defined with a nodular or
masslike appearance, others are less well demarcated and amorphous in character.
Note the very different appearance of BOOP from obliterative bronchiolitis (Figs.
5-9 through 5-12); the latter is characterized by areas of hyperlucent parenchyma
and vasoconstriction.

BOOP is characterized by the presence of granulation tissue within small airways and of areas of organizing pneumonia. It is clinically and pathologically different from bronchiolitis obliterans and usually idiopathic.

The HRCT findings of BOOP are numerous and nonspecific. They include
patchy unilateral or bilateral air-space opacification of a ground-glass or soft-tissue
density, small nodular opacities, irregular linear opacities, bronchial wall thickening
and dilatation, and small pleural effusions. The nodules and air space consolidation
represent different degrees of the same nonspecific inflammatory process that involves the bronchioles, alveolar ducts, and alveoli.[10] HRCT scans depict the
anatomic distribution and extent of BOOP more accurately than chest radiographs.[10]

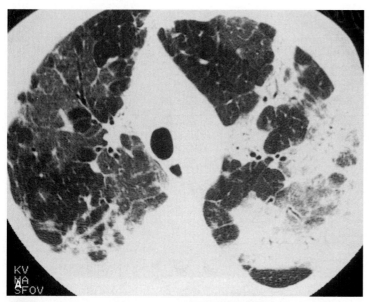

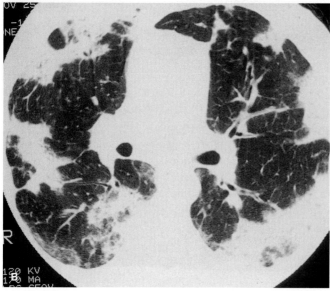

FIGURE 5-16

HRCT scans from this patient with chronic eosinophilic pneumonia show nonspecific diffuse but patchy bilateral regions of opacification.

The classic radiographic pattern of chronic eosinophilic pneumonia is opacification of the air space in the peripheral third of the lungs, often with upper lung zone distribution. However, this classic pattern is seen in only a minority of patients with this disease; more often the areas of opacification are distributed diffusely. The CT pattern, although helpful, is not sufficiently specific for diagnosis and must be correlated with the clinical scenario.[11] A similar, nonspecific peripheral pattern of airspace opacification can be seen with other inflammatory processes of the airways or pulmonary vasculature, including such diverse etiologies as pyogenic pneumonia or pulmonary vasculitides; the clinical scenario is useful in limiting the differential diagnosis.

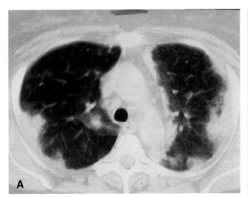
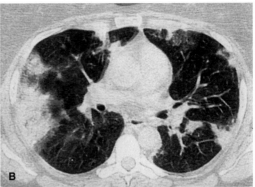

Figure 5-17

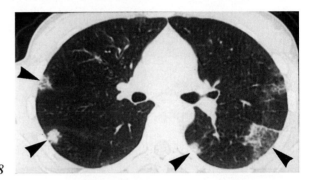

Figure 5-18

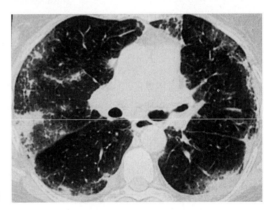

Figure 5-19

FIGURES 5-17, 5-18, and 5-19

HRCT scans from these three patients with chronic eosinophilic pneumonia show multiple diffuse, bilateral, peripheral patchy regions of opacification, some with a nodular appearance (*arrowheads*). There is often an upper lung distribution. Differential diagnostic considerations include BOOP and, in certain situations, reactivation tuberculosis.

When peripheral air space disease is present in chronic eosinophilic pneumonia, it is often better detected with CT than with chest radiographs because of the improved detection of differing degrees of attenuation by the CT hardware coupled with the ability to resolve for overlapping structures. Indeed, by using CT and in particular HRCT, this pattern may be identified in patients whose chest radiographs do not reveal it.

REFERENCES

1. Silver SF, Müller NL, Miller RR, Lefcoe MS. Hypersensitivity pneumonitis: Evaluation with CT. Radiology 1989; 173:441–445

2. Lynch DA, Rose CS, Way D, King TEJ. Hypersensitivity pneumonitis: Sensitivity of high-resolution CT in a population-based study. AJR 1992; 159:469–472

3. Fraser R, Pare J, Pare P, Fraser R, Genereux G. Diagnosis of Diseases of the Chest, 3rd ed. Philadelphia: W.B. Saunders, 1990, pp 1273–1290 and 2058–2059

4. Buschman DL, Gamsu G, Waldron JAJ, Klein JS, King TEJ. Chronic hypersensitivity pneumonitis: Use of CT in diagnosis. AJR 1992; 159:957–960

5. Adler BD, Padley SP, Müller NL, Remy JM, Remy J. Chronic hypersensitivity pneumonitis: High-resolution CT and radiographic features in 16 patients. Radiology 1992; 185:91–95

6. Urbanski SJ, Kossakowska AE, Curtis J, et al. Idiopathic small airways pathology in patients with graft-versus-host disease following allogeneic bone marrow transplantation. Am J Surg Pathol 1987; 11:965–971

7. Sweatman MC, Millar AB, Strickland B, Turner WM. Computed tomography in adult obliterative bronchiolitis. Clin Radiol 1990; 41:116–119

8. Stern EJ, Samples TL. Dynamic ultrafast high resolution CT findings in a case of Swyer-James syndrome. Pediatr Radiol 1992; 22:350–352

9. Webb WR, Stern EJ, Kanth N, Gamsu G. Dynamic pulmonary CT: Findings in healthy adult men. Radiology 1993; 186:117–124

10. Müller NL, Staples CA, Miller RR. Bronchiolitis obliterans organizing pneumonia: CT features in 14 patients. AJR 1990; 154:983–987

11. Mayo JR, Müller NL, Road J, Sisler J, Lillington G. Chronic eosinophilic pneumonia: CT findings in six cases. AJR 1989; 153:727–730

High-Resolution CT of the Chest: Comprehensive Atlas
by Eric J. Stern and Stephen J. Swensen,
Lippincott–Raven Publishers, Philadelphia © 1996.

Cystic Lung Diseases
6

Lymphangioleiomyomatosis
Tuberous sclerosis of the lung
Eosinophilic granuloma of the lung
Histiocytosis X
Juvenile laryngotracheobronchial papillomatosis

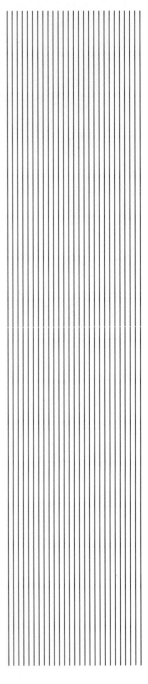

105

Lymphangioleiomyomatosis

MILD DISEASE WITH PNEUMOTHORAX

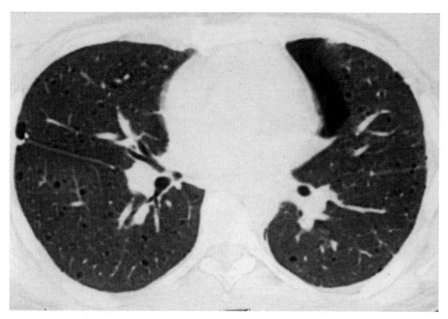

FIGURE 6-1

HRCT scan shows multiple, evenly distributed small cystic spaces, with well-defined walls throughout the lungs, typical for mild lymphangioleiomyomatosis (LAM). Note also the left anteromedial pneumothorax, a common complication of LAM.

LAM is a rare disease of unknown etiology affecting women of reproductive age. Pathologically, LAM is characterized by progressive proliferation of smooth muscle in the airways, arterioles, venules, and lymphatics of the lung, leading to progressive shortness of breath, lung cysts, pneumothorax, hemoptysis, and chylous effusion.

The HRCT and pathologic appearances of LAM are indistinguishable from those of cystic lung disease of tuberous sclerosis. Although pleural effusions are common in LAM, nodules are not seen, unlike in eosinophilic granuloma of the lung.

MODERATE SEVERITY OF DISEASE

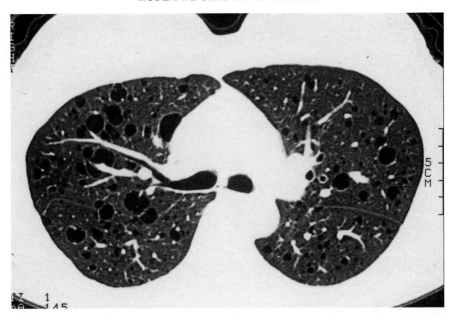

FIGURE 6-2

HRCT scan from a patient with lymphangioleiomyomatosis (LAM) of moderate severity shows cystic spaces that are larger than those in Figure 6-1 but still relatively spherical, with well-defined walls. They are distributed diffusely in the central and peripheral regions of the parenchyma. Although eosinophilic granuloma may also have a predominantly cystic appearance, it is distinguished from LAM by the relative upper zone predominance of cysts, often sparing the lung bases. In LAM the distribution is diffuse and uniform. The "cysts" of eosinophilic granuloma of the lung often are bizarre-shaped and are actually regions of paracicatricial emphysema. The "cysts" in LAM are spherical and usually have a thin but discernible wall. In contrast, the HRCT findings in centrilobular emphysema show lucent regions without discernible walls for the most part (see Figs. 7-2 through 7-4). In LAM the lung parenchyma between the cysts appears normal on high-resolution CT; there are never lung nodules, as in eosinophilic granuloma.

SEVERE DISEASE

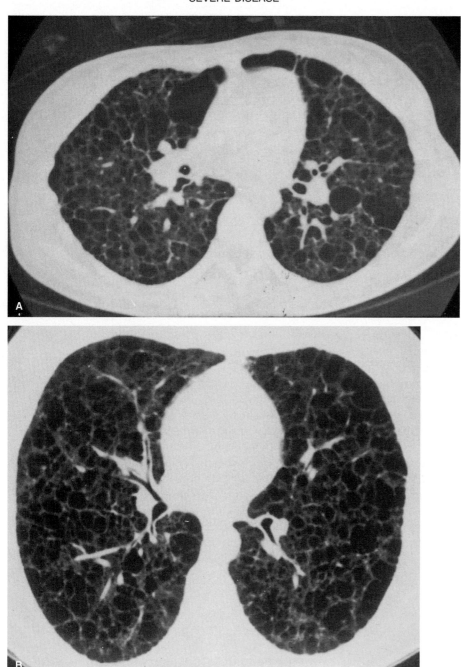

FIGURE 6-3

HRCT scans from two different patients with severe cystic lung disease of lymphangioleiomyomatosis show innumerable cysts ranging from a few millimeters to 5 cm
in diameter.

ZONAL DISTRIBUTION OF DISEASE IN A PATIENT WITH EFFUSION

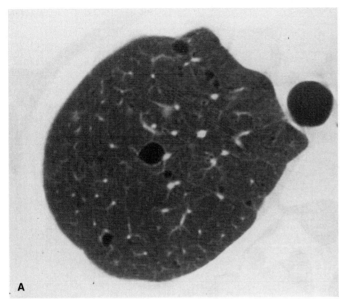

Upper lung zone

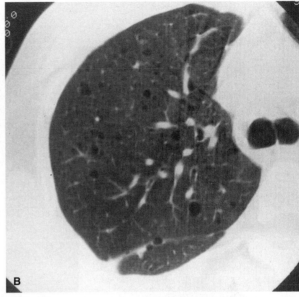

Middle lung zone

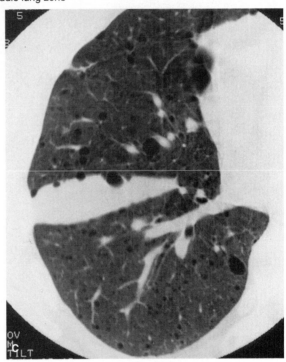

Lower lung zone

FIGURE 6-4

HRCT scans from a patient with mild lymphangioleiomyomatosis show a diffuse, random distribution of cysts of various size. These are distributed throughout all zones of the lungs but predominate in the bases. The cysts have thin discrete walls, unlike in emphysema. Note the effusion in the major fissure—probably chylous.

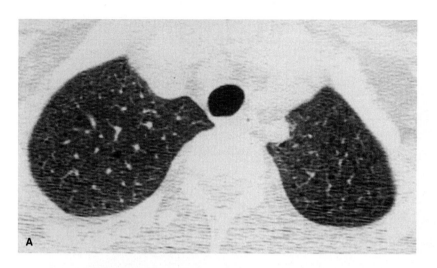

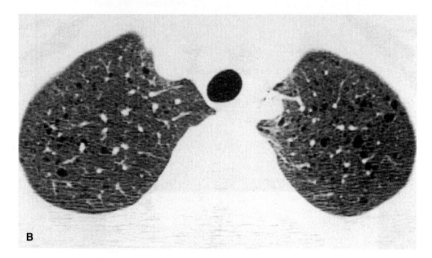

FIGURE 6-5

HRCT scans from a patient with lymphangioleiomyomatosis performed at an interval of 4 months show enlarging and more numerous cysts, indicating progression of the disease. Note the increase in the size and number of typical cysts.

MILD DISEASE

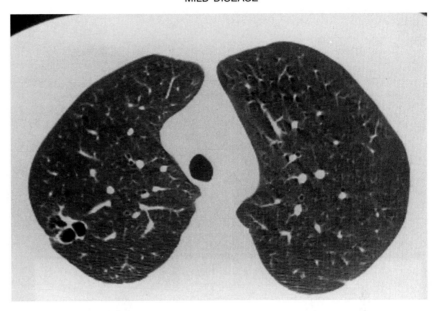

FIGURE 6-6

HRCT scan shows very mild cystic lung disease in a woman with tuberous sclerosis whose disease involved predominantly the brain and kidneys, largely sparing the lungs. At present, it is generally acknowledged that the lung involvement of tuberous sclerosis is indistinguishable from that of lymphangioleiomyomatosis by histologic and HRCT examination.[1]

MODERATE DISEASE

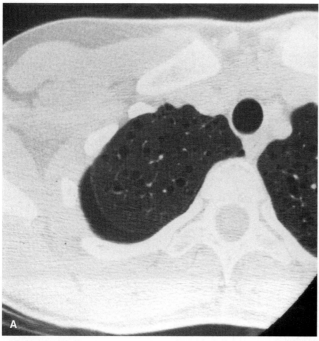

Upper lung zones

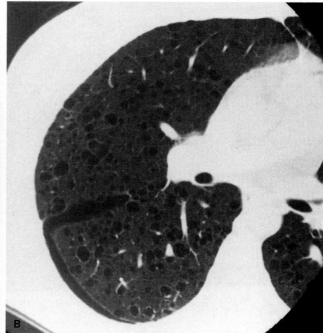

Middle lung zones

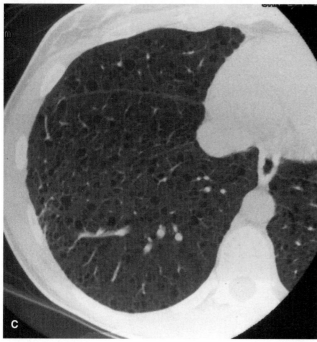

Lower lung zones

FIGURE 6-7

HRCT scans from a woman with tuberous sclerosis shows moderate cystic lung disease. Cysts are distributed diffusely from apex to base in a random pattern. Note the pneumothorax, one of the complications of this disease, and of lymphangioleiomyomatosis.

SEVERE DISEASE

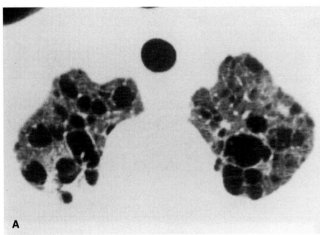

Upper lung zones

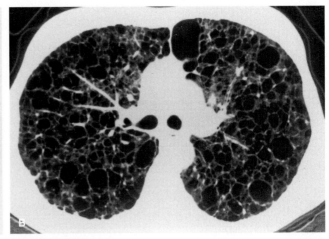

Middle lung zones

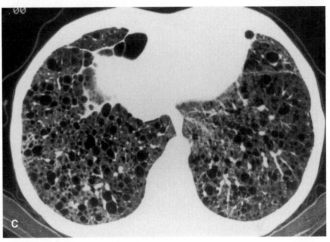

Lower lung zones

FIGURE 6-8

HRCT scans from a woman with tuberous sclerosis show extensive, end-stage cystic lung disease.

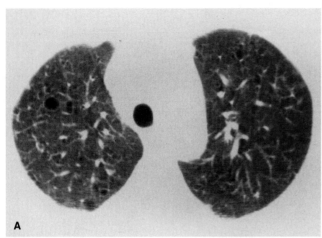

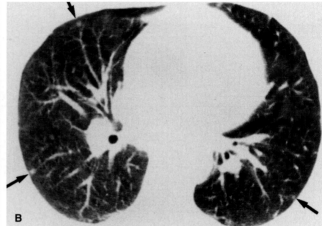

Figure 6-9

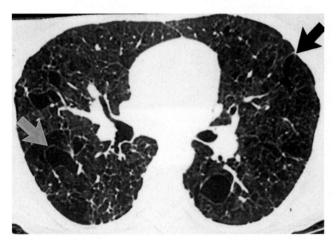

Figure 6-10

FIGURES 6-9 and 6-10

HRCT scans from two different patients with eosinophilic granuloma (EG) of the lung show typical relatively small, thin-walled, bilateral, and symmetric lung cysts. In Figure 6–9A, the cysts involve primarily the upper lobes; in the lower lungs (B) there are no cysts, but small nodules are present (*small arrows*).

Histiocytosis X is a disease of unknown etiology that usually affects multiple organs. The age of onset, the clinical course, and the disease pattern permit a distinction to be made among three types: Letterer-Siwe, Hand-Schüller-Christian, and EG. When the disease process is confined to the lung, usually in adults, it is often referred to as EG of the lung although there is some overlap. EG is more common in Caucasians and most of those affected are cigarette smokers.

HRCT scans can show a variety of patterns of disease in EG. Cysts, nodules, or cysts and nodules may be identified. Cysts are usually less than 10 mm in diameter. Nodules are usually less than 5 mm in diameter. Cysts may attain bizarre or unusual shapes (*large arrows*); the cysts are caused by paracicatricial emphysema. As in lymphangioleiomyomatosis, the interstitial patterns that appear on chest radiographs are actually innumerable overlapping lung cysts. Lung cysts have no central or peripheral distribution, but nodules can be seen in association with the central bronchovascular bundles of secondary lobules.[2]

SEVERE DISEASE WITH COALESCENCE OF APICAL CYSTS

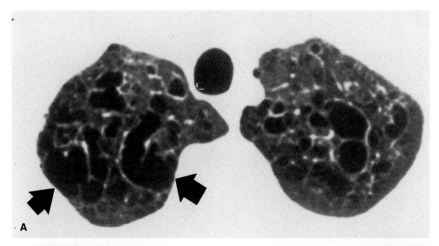

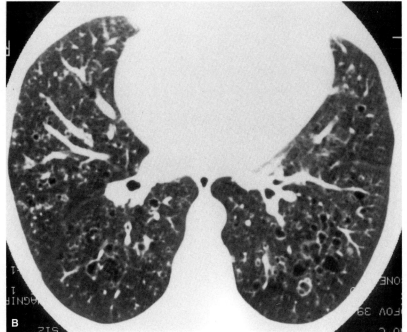

FIGURE 6-11

HRCT scans from this patient with eosinophilic granuloma show lung cysts that are larger and more extensive in the apex, much less severe in the midlung, and absent in the lung bases (not shown). The cysts can attain unusual shapes, perhaps from coalescence of regions of paracicatricial emphysema (*arrows*). No nodules were present in this patient.

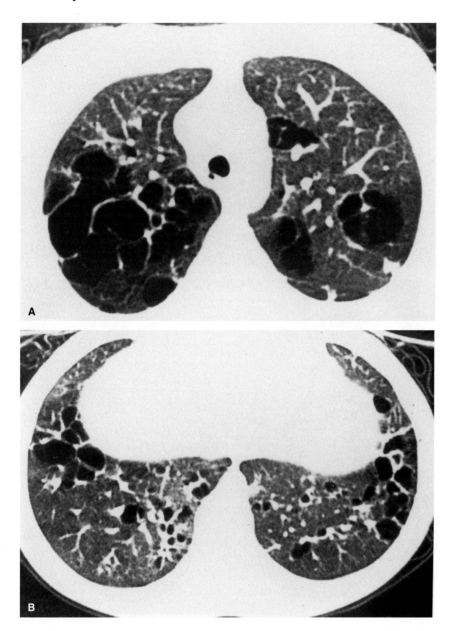

FIGURE 6-12

HRCT scans from this 10-year-old boy with the eosinophilic granuloma form of histiocytosis X show typical features, with apical coalescence of cystic lung disease. In addition, the patient had multiple organ system involvement with diabetes insipidus and a lytic sphenoid bone lesion.

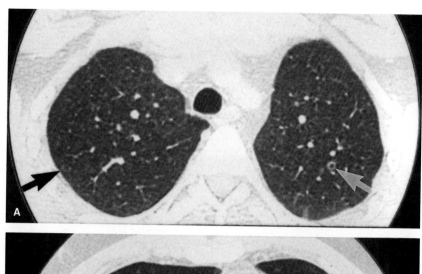

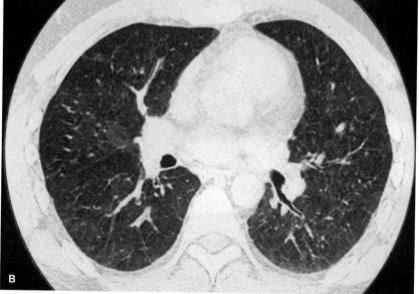

FIGURE 6-13

HRCT scans from this patient with eosinophilic granuloma show diffuse small nodular infiltrates in the upper lungs (A), whereas the lower lungs are relatively spared (B). In the apex of each lung there is a single cyst (*arrows*). In the apices, the nodules are diffusely disseminated without central, peripheral, or bronchovascular distribution.

This apical distribution of the nodules and the presence of cysts suggest the possibility of eosinophilic granuloma. Differential diagnosis includes sarcoidosis, granulomatous infection, and hematogenous metastases. In eosinophilic granuloma, HRCT can show a variety of patterns of disease, including lung cysts only, the combination of cysts and nodules, or predominantly nodules only, as in this case.

Juvenile laryngotracheobronchial papillomatosis

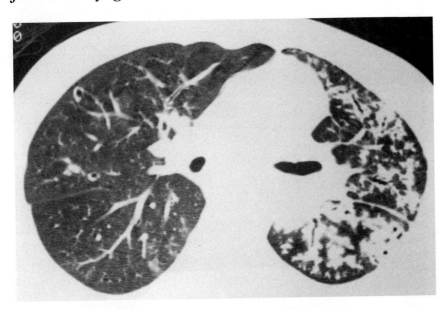

FIGURE 6-14

HRCT scan in a patient with juvenile laryngotracheobronchial papillomatosis shows multiple, small, solid and cavitary/cystic nodules throughout the lower lungs, worse in the left lung. The lesions tend to be centered within the bronchovascular bundles.

Juvenile laryngotracheobronchial papillomatosis is a recurrent, prolonged disease usually confined to the upper airway. Pulmonary involvement is present in only 1% of patients with this infection and carries a poor prognosis. The lung lesions appear either cystic or solid and represent benign squamous cell proliferations or papillomas with or without central cavities containing debris or air. Papillomas may spread from the larynx to the bronchi and bronchioles. This occurs by direct extension, lesions developing in the lungs many years after the onset of laryngeal papillomatosis. Whereas the laryngeal lesions may regress spontaneously, it is uncommon for the lung lesions to do so. Lung cancer has been reported to occur with increased frequency in these patients.[3]

REFERENCES

1. Webb WR, Müller NL, Naidich DP. High-Resolution CT of the Lung. New York: Raven Press, 1992, p 116

2. Moore AD, Godwin JD, Müller NL, et al. Pulmonary histiocytosis X: Comparison of radiographic and CT findings. Radiology 1989; 172:249–254

3. Kramer SS, Wehunt WD, Stocker JT, Kashima H. Pulmonary manifestations of juvenile laryngotracheal papillomatosis. AJR 1985; 144:687–694

High-Resolution CT of the Chest: Comprehensive Atlas
by Eric J. Stern and Stephen J. Swensen,
Lippincott–Raven Publishers, Philadelphia © 1996.

Obstructive Lung Diseases

7

Panlobular emphysema

Centrilobular emphysema

Fibrosis associated with centrilolobular emphysema

Superior segment centrilolobular emphysema

Asymmetric emphysema

Focal asymmetric centrilolobular emphysema

Apparent asymmetric emphysema

Paraseptal (distal lobular) emphysema

Paraseptal emphysema—spectrum of severity

Atypical bullous emphysema

Giant bullous emphysema (vanishing lung syndrome)

Paracicatricial emphysema

Intralobar sequestration

Extralobar bronchopulmonary sequestration

Bronchogenic cyst

Congenital lobar emphysema

Micronodular opacities in cigarette smoker's lung

Ground-glass opacities in cigarette smoker's lung

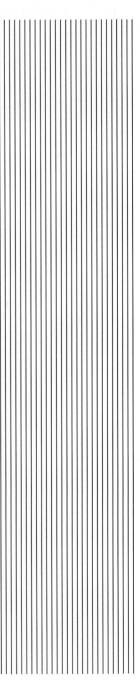

Panlobular emphysema

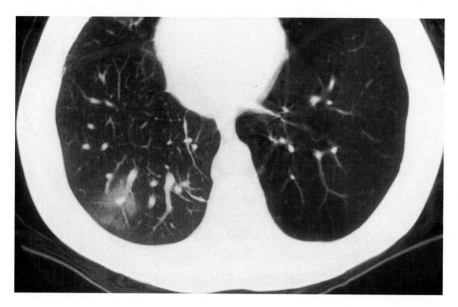

FIGURE 7-1

HRCT scan from a woman who received a right lung transplant for alpha$_1$-antiprotease deficiency shows diffuse low attenuation and thinned out vascular structures in the native left lung. This appearance of diffuse low attenuation lung parenchyma is typical of panlobular emphysema.

Four different morphologic subtypes of emphysema have been described: panlobular, centrilobular, paraseptal (also called distal lobular), and paracicatricial (irregular or scar). As the terms imply, emphysema within the secondary pulmonary lobule can be a diffuse lobular process, as in panlobular emphysema, or it may be locally selective with proximal (centrilobular) or peripheral (distal lobular) lobular involvement.

Panlobular emphysema characteristically has a lower lobe distribution, although it can occur anywhere in the lung. Panlobular emphysema is seen with alpha$_1$-antiprotease (antitrypsin) deficiency and in obliterative bronchiolitis. In smokers, panlobular emphysema can be seen, in conjunction with centrilobular emphysema, but it is not the dominant morphologic abnormality and is probably just advanced centrilobular emphysema. Panlobular emphysema may also be a normal senescent finding in nonsmokers.[1]

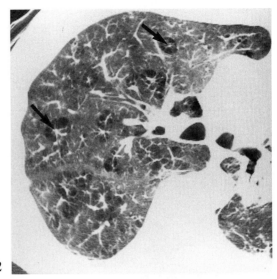

Figure 7-2

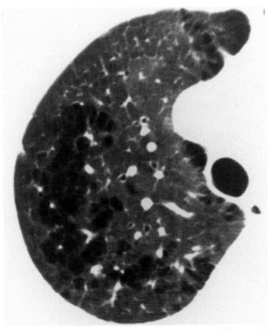

Figure 7-3

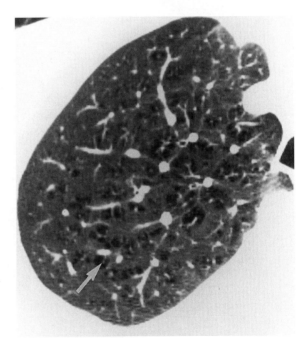

Figure 7-4

FIGURES 7-2, 7-3, and 7-4

HRCT scans from three patients with centrilobular emphysema show multiple focal rounded lucencies of various size (ranging from 5 to 10 mm), surrounded by normal parenchyma, without discrete walls. Note the small white dots in the center of these lucencies, which are the preserved centrilobular core structures (*arrows*). The appearance of a partial "wall" may be seen when an emphysematous space abuts a vessel, usually a vein.

The most common form of emphysema is centrilobular emphysema. Strongly associated with cigarette smoking, centrilobular emphysema results from destruction of alveoli surrounding the proximal respiratory bronchioles. This disease has a predilection for the upper lung zones, including the apical and posterior segments of the upper lobes and the superior segments of the lower lobes.[2]

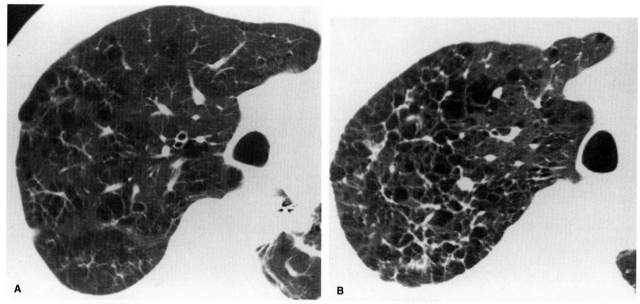

Figure 7-5

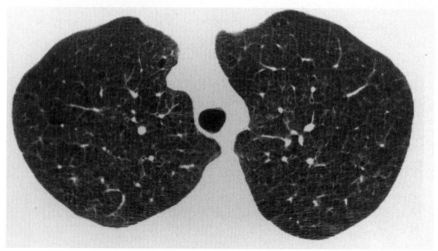

Figure 7-6

FIGURES 7-5 and 7-6

HRCT scans from two cigarette smokers. The caudal regions of the right upper lobe (Fig. 7-5A) show areas of typical centrilobular emphysema whose walls are characteristically undefinable. By contrast, in the more apical regions of the same lobe (Fig. 7-5B) the emphysematous spaces have discrete walls that are thicker than normal interlobular septa or other linear pulmonary structures. Similar findings of fibrosis associated with centrilobular emphysema are noted in Figure 7-6. Because cigarette smoking causes inflammation at the terminal bronchiole and alveolar levels, fibrosis can coexist with emphysema, although it may be difficult to detect on radiographic or even CT images. Rarely, this appearance may be confused with eosinophilic granuloma of the lung (see Figs. 6-11 and 6-12).

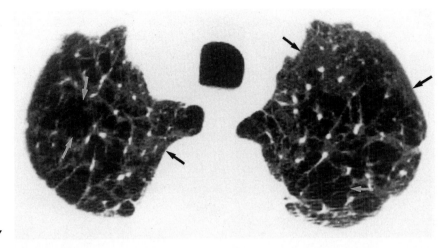

Figure 7-7

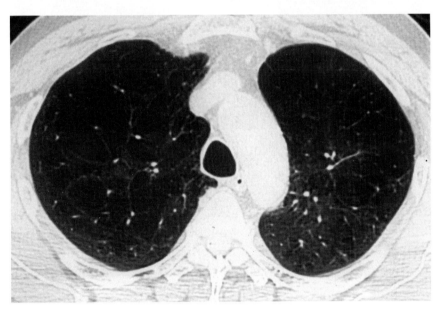

Figure 7-8

FIGURES 7-7 and 7-8

CT scans from two patients with long cigarette smoking histories show severe bilateral centrilobular emphysema in the upper lobes. Note multiple well-defined confluent lucencies (*white arrows*), most without defined margins, surrounded by patchy areas of more normal-appearing parenchyma (*black arrows*). The confluent areas of low attenuation lung parenchyma probably represent areas of panlobular emphysema as well as centrilobular emphysema.

When severe, centrilobular emphysema can involve the entire lobule and appear similar to panlobular emphysema; there is much more extensive lung destruction. However, pathologically, the dominant form of emphysema is centrilobular.

When any emphysematous space is larger than 1 cm, it can be defined as a bulla.[3]

Superior segment centrilobular emphysema

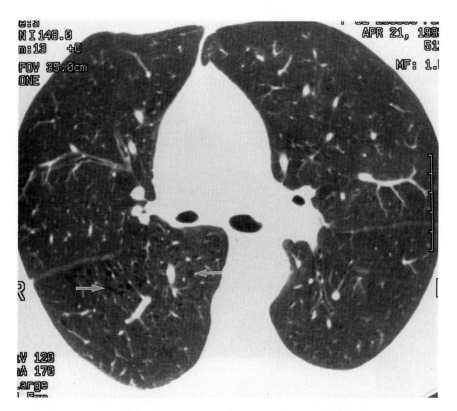

FIGURE 7-9

HRCT scan shows mild centrilobular emphysema in the superior segments of the lower lobes. Centrilobular emphysema has a predilection for the upper portion of the individual lobes, i.e., the apical and posterior segments of the upper lobes, and for the superior segments of the lower lobes,[2] as in this patient.

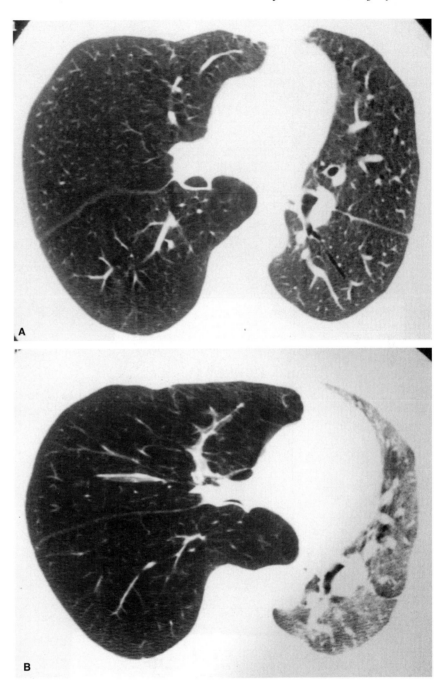

FIGURE 7-10

Inspiration (A) and expiration (B) HRCT scans show asymmetric emphysema of the right lung, in this case secondary to a left lung transplant. The normal exit of air from the left lung causes a shift of the mediastinum to the left. Severe emphysematous changes in the right lung produce overinflation. The expiratory image reveals air trapping in the right lung.

Focal asymmetric centrilobular emphysema

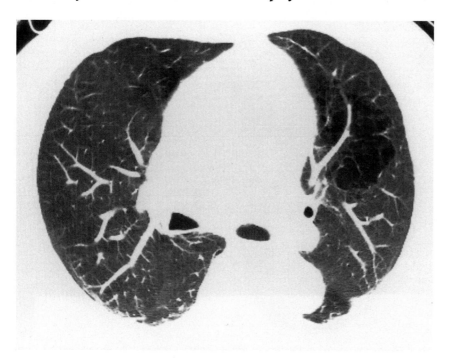

FIGURE 7-11

HRCT scan shows an isolated area of low attenuation in the lingula, an unusual focal region of asymmetric centrilobular emphysema.

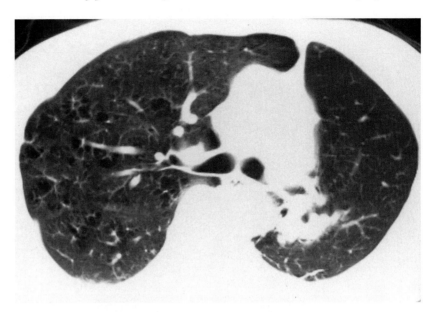

FIGURE 7-12

HRCT scan shows apparent asymmetric centrilobular emphysema involving the right lung only. However, this patient (a cigarette smoker) has undergone left upper lobectomy, and thus the left hemithorax is filled by the overinflated hyperlucent left lower lobe and lingula, regions of lung with no detectable centrilobular emphysema.

Paraseptal (distal lobular) emphysema

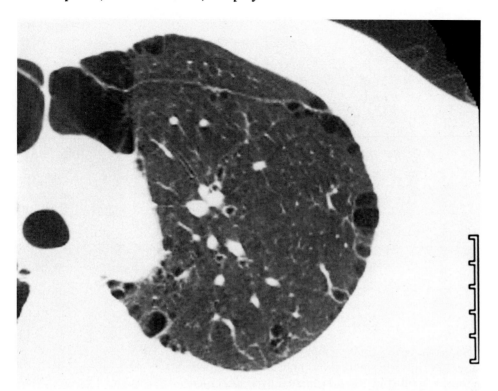

FIGURE 7-13

Small lucencies (usually <1 cm) occupy the subpleural location. These are typical of paraseptal emphysema and should not be confused with cystic lung disease.

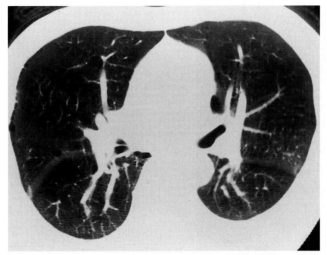

Mild   *Figure 7-14*

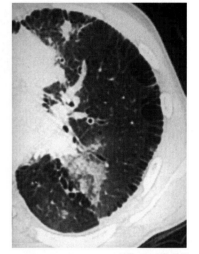

Moderate   *Figure 7-15*

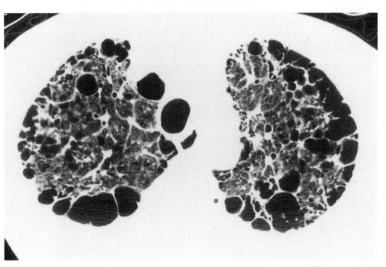

Severe   *Figure 7-16*

FIGURES 7-14, 7-15, and 7-16

HRCT scans from three patients show the spectrum of pulmonary involvement that may result from paraseptal emphysema, typically <1 cm peripheral lucencies, often with well-circumscribed borders. This form of emphysema may be focal or multifocal and has a predilection for the fissures and sharp pleural reflections.

The cause of this form of emphysema is unknown, and can develop in young individuals who are otherwise normal. It is unassociated with air flow obstruction or chronic clinical symptoms, but may coexist with centrilobular emphysema, as is shown in the example of severe paraseptal emphysema (Fig. 7-16).

Coalescence of this type of emphysema, from unknown influences, is generally regarded as a mechanism of bullae and giant bullae formation (vanishing lung syndrome).[4] Paraseptal emphysema appears to be important in the development of spontaneous pneumothoraces.[5,6]

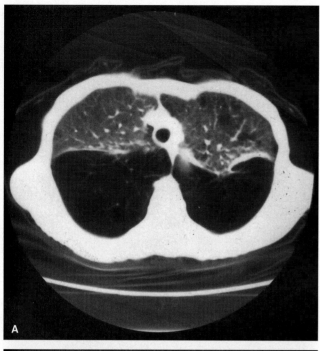

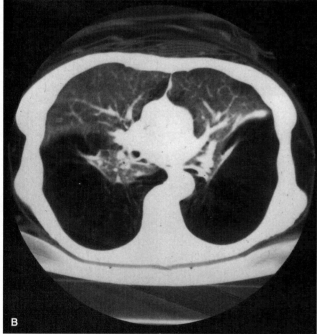

FIGURE 7-17

HRCT scans show a distinctly unusual case of bullous emphysema with a posterior distribution. The cause of this peculiar distribution of bullae is unknown.

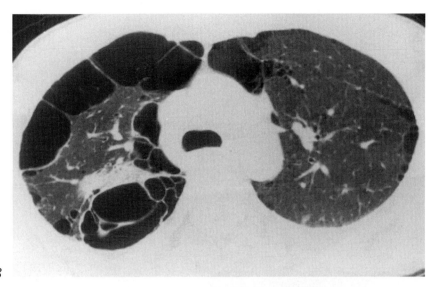

Figure 7-18

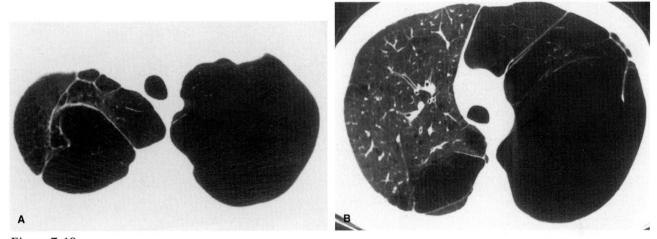

Figure 7-19

FIGURES 7-18 and 7-19

HRCT scans from two young dyspneic patients show extensive lung destruction with multiple large bullae occupying the hemithoraces. Note the marked asymmetry. In Figure 7-18, the more normal-appearing lung shows paraseptal emphysema in the left lung, whereas in Figure 7-19 there is minimal intraparenchymal centrilobular emphysema anteromedially in the right lung.

These findings are typical of idiopathic giant bullous emphysema, also called vanishing lung syndrome. This is a severe, precocious, giant bullous emphysema in the upper lungs, often asymmetric, found in cigarette smoking young dyspneic men. The syndrome also can be seen in nonsmokers. The dominant and consistent HRCT feature in both smokers and nonsmokers is that of extensive paraseptal emphysema coalescing into the giant bullae.[7]

Paracicatricial emphysema

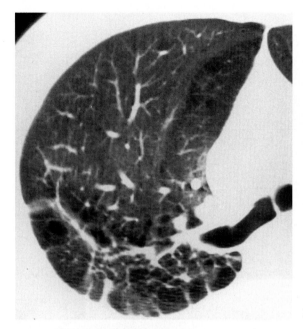

Figure 7-20

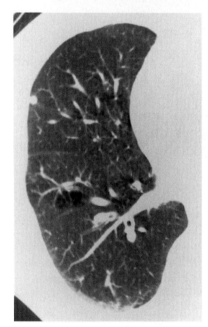

Figure 7-21

FIGURES 7-20 and 7-21

HRCT images from two different patients depict focal areas of low attenuation surrounding obvious irregular linear opacities that represent scars.

Paracicatricial emphysema (also called irregular or scar emphysema) may develop in any part of the lobule. It is always associated with adjacent fibrosis that may be focal (e.g., apical scarring of old granulomatous disease) or diffuse (progressive massive fibrosis caused by silicosis). However, the emphysematous changes usually are of no functional or clinical significance; the "cystic" changes seen in eosinophilic granulomatosis are also caused by paracicatricial emphysema (see Figs. 6-9 through 6-12).

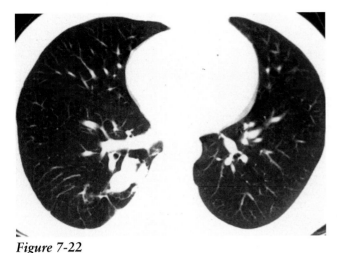

Figure 7-22

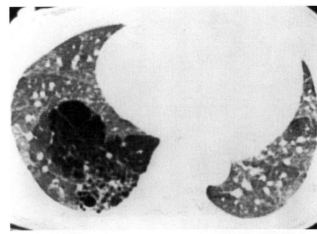

Figure 7-23

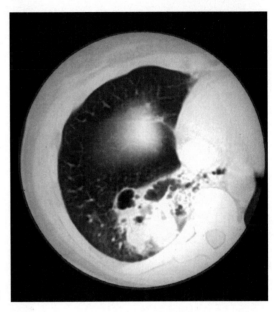

Figure 7-24

FIGURES 7-22, 7-23, and 7-24

HRCT scans from three different patients each show a multicystic mass centered in the posterior basal segment of the right lower lobe. The location and appearance are typical of intralobar sequestration, a malformation of controversial etiology consisting of nonfunctioning, abnormal lung tissue contained within otherwise normal lung tissue.

A bronchopulmonary sequestration is probably a congenital anomaly in which a portion of lung develops abnormally and without normal or direct continuity to the tracheobronchial tree. Such sequestered regions of lung always receive systemic arterial supply, often from anomalous vessels that arise below the diaphragm. Sequestrations are further classified as intralobar or extralobar types. Intralobar sequestrations drain into the pulmonary venous system, do not have a separate pleural investment, are usually aerated, and appear in childhood or adulthood, whereas extralobar sequestrations drain systemically, have a separate pleural investment, are not aerated and are therefore more masslike, and often appear during infancy. Extralobular sequestrations are most often identified in the left lower lobe adjacent to the diaphragm.

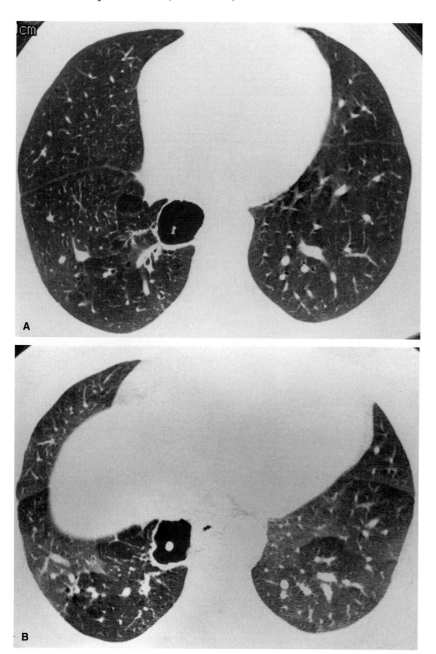

FIGURE 7-25

Inspiration and expiration HRCT scans show a nonsegmental area in the right lower lobe containing multiple cysts and low attenuation parenchyma typical of an intralobar sequestration. The lucency of the surrounding lung is a particular characteristic of intralobar sequestrations.[8]

Intralobar bronchopulmonary sequestrations lack normal communications with the tracheobronchial tree; however, they can be ventilated by collateral air drift or through fistulous bronchial communications, as suggested by the air trapping at expiration HRCT.

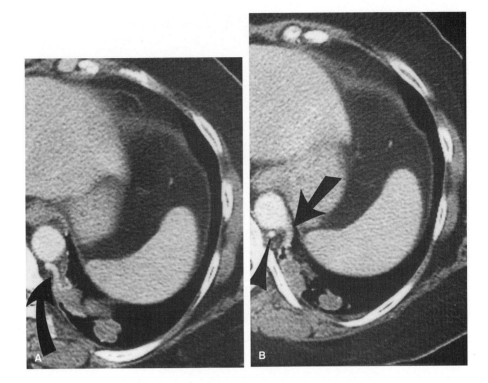

FIGURE 7-26

Enhanced CT scans show a mass in the posterior basal segment of the left lower lobe. Note the systemic artery extending into the mass from the descending thoracic aorta (*arrow*) and the systemic vein (*curved arrow*) extending from the mass into the hemiazygos vein (*arrowhead*). These findings are diagnostic of an extralobar bronchopulmonary sequestration.

Bronchogenic cyst

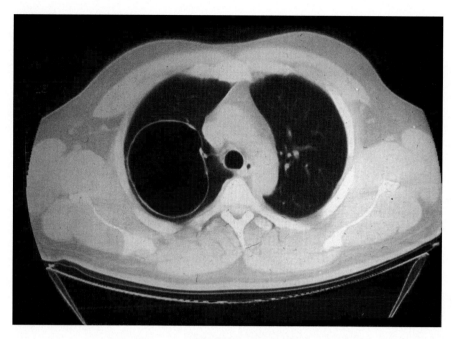

FIGURE 7-27

CT scan from a patient with a large cystic lucency in the right upper lobe. The smooth thin wall is typical of a bronchogenic cyst.

Bronchogenic cysts are one form of bronchopulmonary foregut duplication cysts. Because communication with the tracheobronchial tree is rare, the contents of the cyst are usually of water density. A rim of calcification may be identified in the wall of some cysts.

Two thirds of the bronchogenic cysts are located in the mediastinum; these are usually in close proximity to the carina, mainstem bronchi, trachea, esophagus, or pericardium. However, up to one third may be located within pulmonary parenchyma or in the inferior pulmonary ligament.[9]

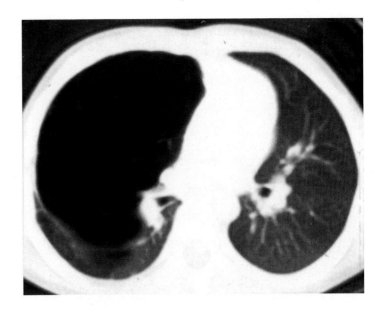

FIGURE 7-28

CT scan from a 3-year-old boy with congenital lobar emphysema of the right upper lobe shows marked hyperinflation with contralateral mediastinal shift and compression of the right lower lobe. The parenchyma of the right upper lobe is almost completely destroyed, and the remaining tissue was collapsed by the marked hyperinflation.

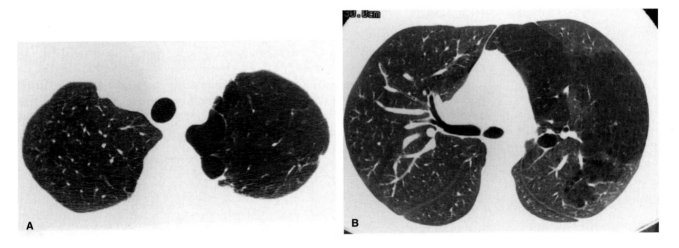

FIGURE 7-29

HRCT scan from a nonsmoking young adult shows multiple well-demarcated regions of low attenuation in the left upper lobe with minimal bullous change at the apex. This was presumed to represent congenital lobar emphysema. Note the sharp transition from emphysematous to normal lung in the lingula.

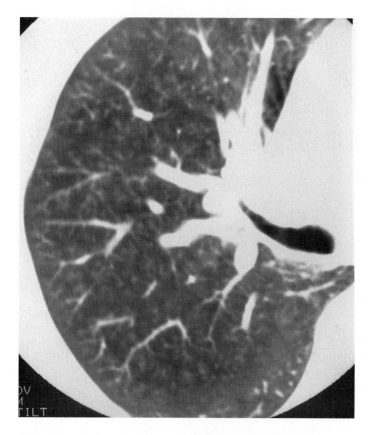

FIGURE 7-30

HRCT scan through the right upper lobe shows multiple subtle ill-defined centrilobular micronodules throughout the parenchyma. These were limited to the upper lobes in this patient.

Cigarette smoking causes a nonspecific inflammatory reaction at the level of the respiratory bronchioles. This reaction includes peribronchiolar fibrosis in some patients. HRCT in cigarette smokers with respiratory bronchiolitis can show subtle, ill-defined centrilobular micronodules that correspond histopathologically to bronchiolectasis and peribronchiolar fibrosis.

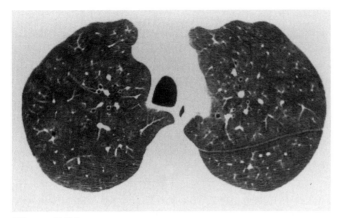

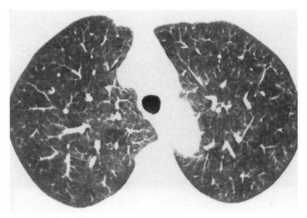

Figure 7-31

Figure 7-32

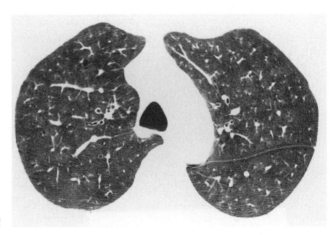

Figure 7-33

FIGURES 7-31, 7-32, and 7-33

HRCT scans from three patients with smoking-related respiratory bronchiolitis show multiple ill-defined, sublobular, nodular ground-glass opacities. There is no evidence of emphysema.

Pathologic studies have revealed that cigarette smoking leads to the accumulation of pigmented macrophages and mucus in the alveolar spaces, mild interstitial inflammation or fibrosis, and bronchiolectasis with peribronchiolar fibrosis.[10] These pathologic features have the above HRCT manifestations.

REFERENCES

1. Anderson AJ, Furlaneto J, Foraker A. Bronchopulmonary derangements in non-smokers. Am Rev Respir Dis 1970; 101:518

2. Fraser R, Pare J, Pare P, Fraser R, Genereux G. Diagnosis of Diseases of the Chest, 3rd ed. Philadelphia: W.B. Saunders, 1990.

3. Tuddenham WJ. Glossary of terms for thoracic radiology: Recommendations of the Nomenclature Committee of the Fleischner Society. AJR 1984; 143:509–517

4. Gaensler E, Jederlinic P, FitzGerald M. Patient work-up for bullectomy. J Thorac Imaging 1986;75–93

5. Bense L, Lewander R, Eklund G, Hedenstierna G, Wiman LG. Nonsmoking, non-alpha 1-antitrypsin deficiency-induced emphysema in nonsmokers with healed spontaneous pneumothorax, identified by computed tomography of the lungs. Chest 1993; 103: 433–438

6. Lesur O, Delorme N, Fromaget JM, Bernadac P, Polu JM. Computed tomography in the etiologic assessment of idiopathic spontaneous pneumothorax. Chest 1990; 98:341–347

7. Stern EJ, Webb WR, Weinacker A, Müller NL. Idiopathic giant bullous emphysema (vanishing lung syndrome): Imaging findings in nine patients. AJR 1994; 162:279–282

8. Stern EJ, Webb WR, Warnock ML, Salmon CJ. Bronchopulmonary sequestration: Dynamic, ultrafast, high-resolution CT evidence of air trapping. AJR 1991; 157:947–949

9. Di LM, Collin PP, Vaillancourt R, Duranceau A. Bronchogenic cysts. J Pediatr Surg 1989; 24:988–991

10. Remy-Jardin M, Remy J, Gosselin B, Becette V, Edme JL. Lung parenchymal changes secondary to cigarette smoking: Pathologic-CT correlations. Radiology 1993; 186:643–651

High-Resolution CT of the Chest: Comprehensive Atlas
by Eric J. Stern and Stephen J. Swensen,
Lippincott–Raven Publishers, Philadelphia © 1996.

Fibrotic Lung Diseases

8

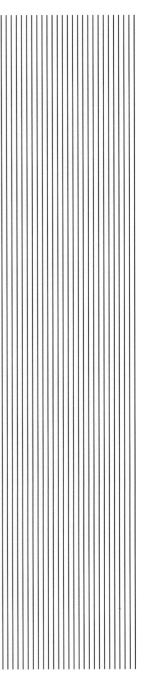

Usual interstitial pneumonia

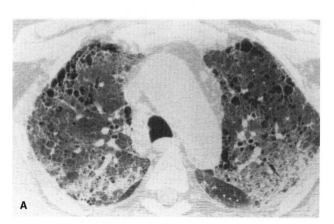

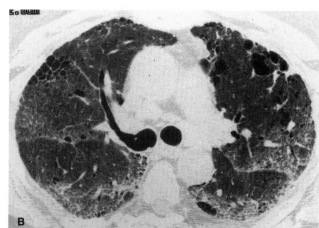

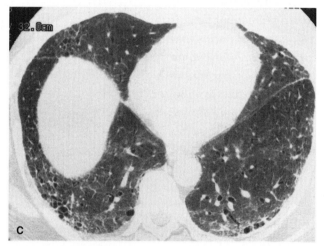

Figure 8-1

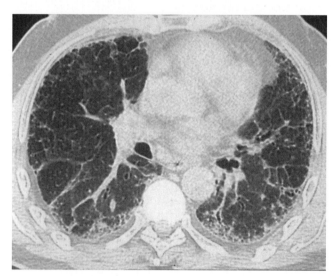

Figure 8-2

FIGURES 8-1 and 8-2

HRCT scans from two patients with typical usual interstitial pneumonia show the characteristic findings of a reticular infiltrative process, architectural distortion, and honeycombing in a peripheral distribution. Usual interstitial pneumonia usually is more profuse at the lung bases. In later stages there are cicatricial changes that may result in traction bronchiectasis and bronchiolectasis. When seen on HRCT, this pattern should be called usual interstitial pneumonia; idiopathic pulmonary fibrosis is a clinical diagnosis. The HRCT pattern of usual interstitial pneumonia is nonspecific and is seen in patients with idiopathic pulmonary fibrosis, asbestosis, and many connective tissue diseases involving the lungs (e.g., rheumatoid arthritis, scleroderma).

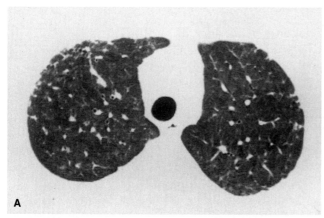

Upper lung zone

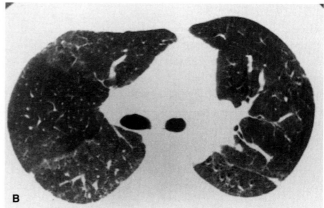

Middle lung zone

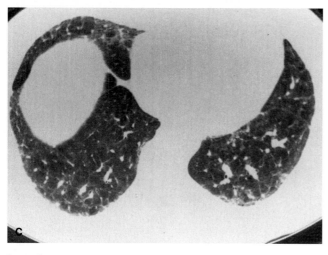

Lower lung zone

Figure 8-3

FIGURES 8-3 and 8-4

HRCT scans from two patients with usual interstitial pneumonia show hazy ground-glass opacities in a peripheral distribution. This pattern may indicate active alveolitis as opposed to burned-out fibrosis and is associated with a better prognosis. Note the typical peripheral and basilar distribution of this infiltrative process. Ground-glass opacity is indicative of active disease only when there is no associated fibrosis, including bronchiectasis or bronchiolectasis. If the ground-glass opacity is associated with signs of architectural distortion, it is probably irreversible and due to fibrosis.[1] Clinically, these patients had idiopathic pulmonary fibrosis.

(continued)

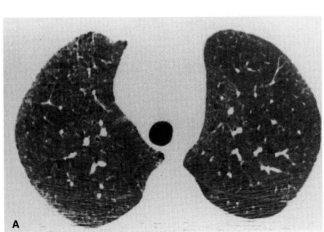

Upper lung zone

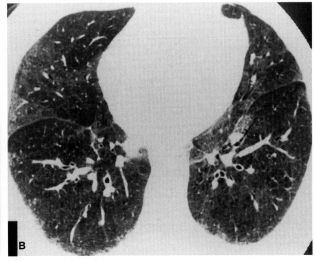

Middle lung zone

Figure 8-4

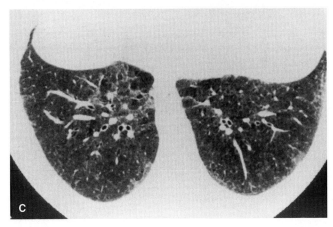

Lower lung zone

FIGURES 8-3 and 8-4 *(continued)*

Mild pulmonary fibrosis

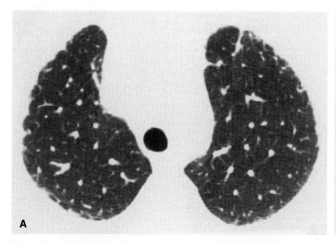

Upper lung zone

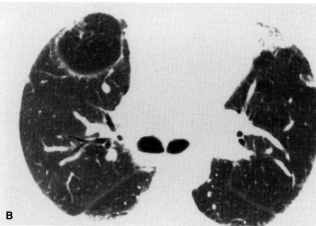

Middle lung zone

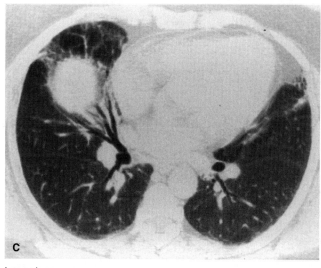

Lower lung zone

Figure 8-5

FIGURES 8-5, 8-6, and 8-7

HRCT scans from these three patients with mild pulmonary fibrosis of unknown etiology—idiopathic pulmonary fibrosis—show mild scarring in a typical peripheral even distribution from apex to base. It is important to note these changes in nondependent regions of the lung, as atelectasis in dependent lung can mimic these mild changes of fibrosis. Obtain scans in the prone position as needed to distinguish the two conditions (see Figs. 14-6 through 14-8).

(continued)

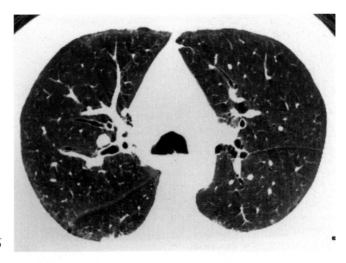

Figure 8-6

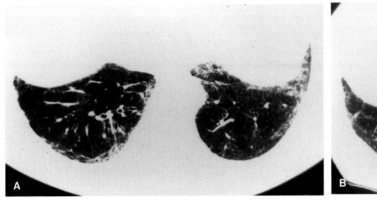
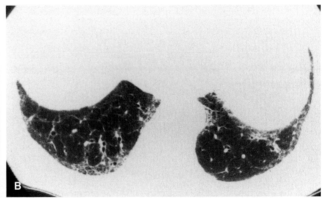

Figure 8-7

FIGURES 8-5, 8-6, and 8-7 *(continued)*

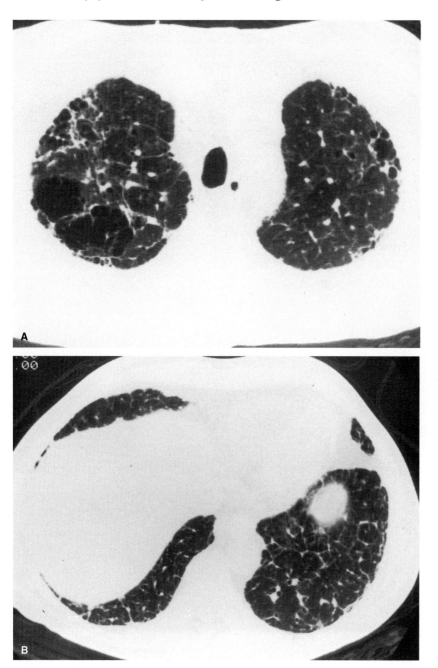

FIGURE 8-8

In addition to typical peripheral fibrosis (B), HRCT scans from this patient with idiopathic pulmonary fibrosis show cystic changes in both upper lobes (A). The etiology of these cysts is unclear. Some may be related to direct alveolar destruction from the inflammatory process and subsequent scarring, whereas others may represent dilated, bronchiolectatic airways.[2]

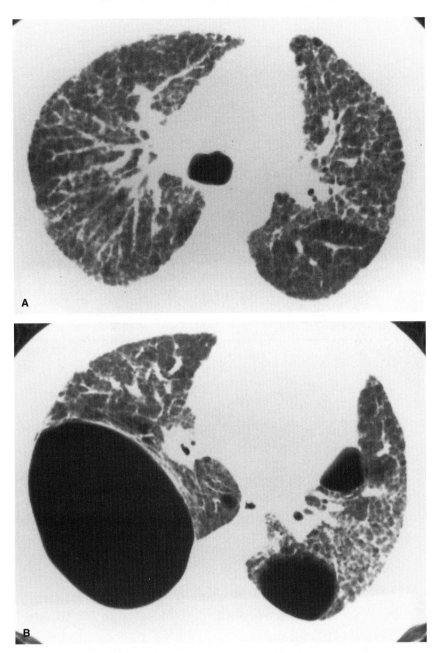

FIGURE 8-9

HRCT scans in this patient with idiopathic pulmonary fibrosis show a somewhat atypical pattern; the fibrosis does not have a peripheral pattern but is more diffuse throughout the parenchyma (A). Also unusual in this case are several large cysts seen at the lung bases (B).

Advanced pulmonary fibrosis

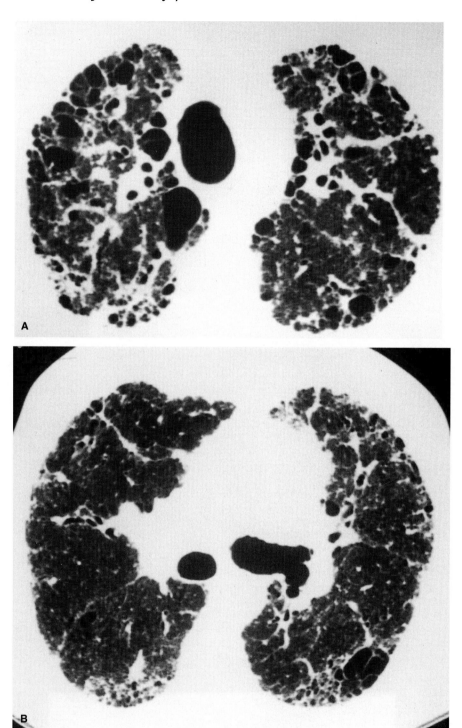

FIGURE 8-10

HRCT scans from this patient with advanced idiopathic pulmonary fibrosis show severe honeycombing and traction dilatation of the trachea and main bronchi. Peripheral honeycombing can have a cystic appearance, but in this case there is extensive architectural distortion not usually associated with cystic lung diseases (see Figs. 6-7 and 6-8).

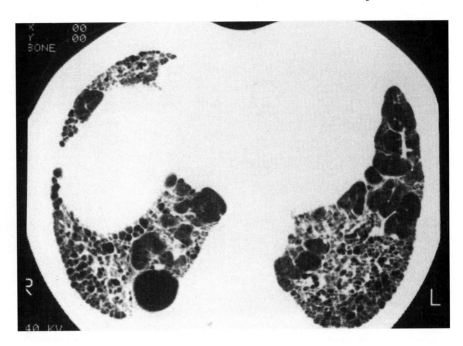

FIGURE 8-11

HRCT scan shows typical end-stage pulmonary fibrosis, in this case caused by giant cell interstitial pneumonia. Giant cell interstitial pneumonia is a distinctive and uncommon form of interstitial pneumonia distinguished by the prominence of large, actively phagocytic alveolar giant cells of histiocytic origin in the presence of chronic interstitial pneumonia. The multinucleated cells lack viral intranuclear inclusions of the type seen in measles pneumonia. Giant cell interstitial pneumonia may be idiopathic or it may occur with occupational exposure to hard metals or cobalt. Hard metal is a mixture of tungsten carbide and cobalt, to which small amounts of other metals may be added. It is widely used for industrial purposes whenever extreme hardness and high temperature resistance are needed, such as for cutting tools, oil well drilling bits, and jet engine exhaust ports. Cobalt is the component of hard metal that can be hazardous. Adverse pulmonary reactions to hard metal include asthma, hypersensitivity pneumonitis, and interstitial fibrosis.[3]

Desquamative interstitial pneumonia

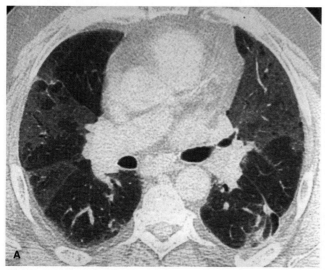
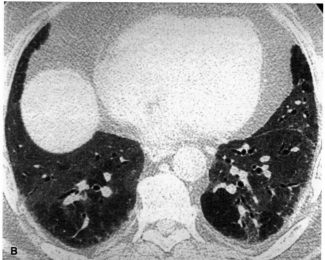

Figure 8-12

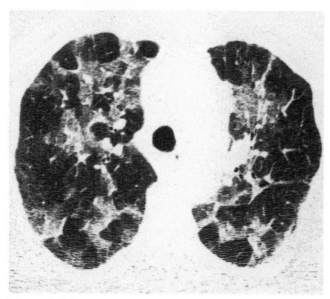

Figure 8-13

FIGURES 8-12 and 8-13

HRCT scans from two patients with desquamative interstitial pneumonia (DIP) show patchy ground-glass opacities. The ground-glass opacities in Figure 8-12 are associated with some architectural distortion (e.g., mild traction bronchiectasis) and therefore probably indicative of fibrosis (implying an irreversible process). The ground-glass opacities in Figure 8-13 have no associated architectural distortion and are consistent with an active, cellular alveolitis.[4] DIP is a distinct form of interstitial pneumonia characterized by a more benign clinical course and specific morphologic and cellular cytologic features. Without treatment, median survival in DIP is over 10 years, whereas in usual interstitial pneumonia it is between 3 and 5 years.[5]

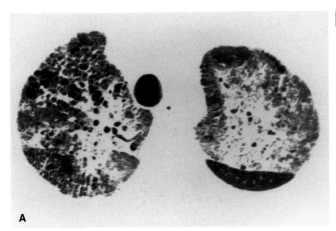

A

Upper lung zone

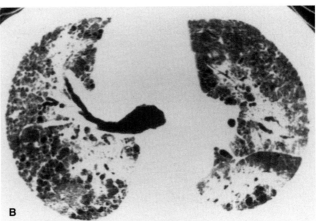

B

Middle lung zone

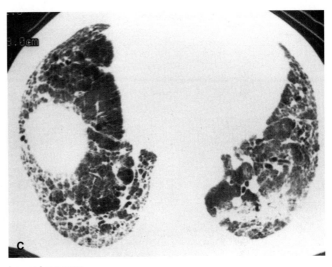

C

Lower lung zone

FIGURE 8-14

HRCT scans from a patient with prior adult respiratory distress syndrome (ARDS) (6 months after acute respiratory failure) show diffuse and extensive honeycombing (lung fibrosis) in the upper and lower, central, and peripheral lung zones. Adult respiratory distress syndrome is a syndrome of diffuse alveolar damage that results in acute respiratory failure and profound hypoxemia. In survivors of ARDS, the lungs frequently progress to a chronic phase (>2 weeks) of alveolar cell hyperplasia, fibroblast proliferation, interstitial collagen deposition, and architectural remodeling. The lung heals with a variable amount of residual fibrosis, severe in this case, over a 6 to 12 month period.

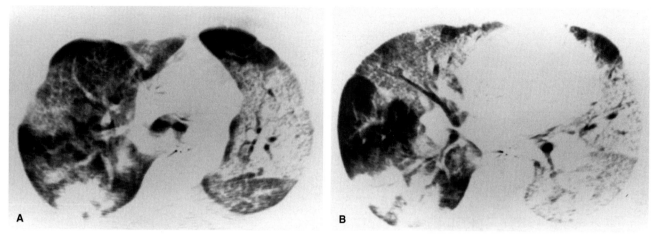

Figure 8-15

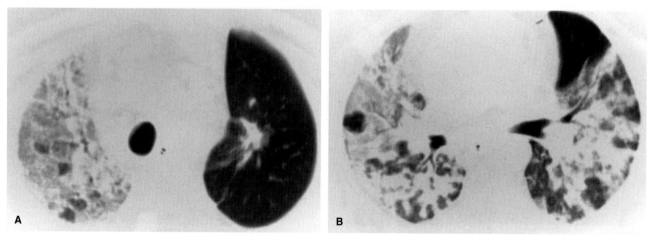

Figure 8-16

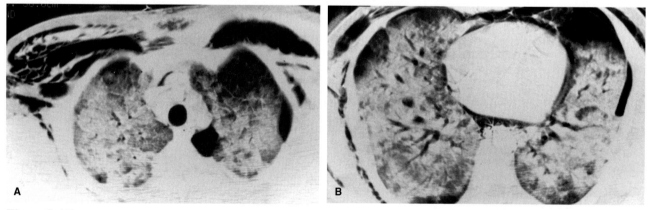

Figure 8-17

FIGURES 8-15, 8-16, and 8-17

CT scans from three different patients in the subacute stage of ARDS show the heterogeneity and patchiness of this syndrome of "diffuse alveolar damage." Note the extensive barotrauma in Figure 8-17.

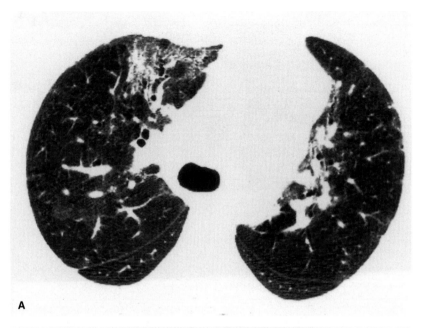

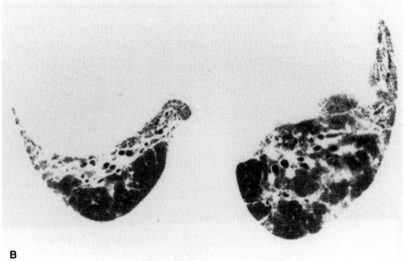

FIGURE 8-18

HRCT scans show many of the typical features of interstitial lung disease associated with collagen vascular disease, in this case rheumatoid lung disease. There is pulmonary fibrosis at the lung bases, secondary traction bronchiectasis, and an area of patchy ground-glass attenuation. Interstitial lung disease is a frequent manifestation of rheumatoid arthritis. Note that the appearance is very similar to that of idiopathic pulmonary fibrosis. The final common pathway of lung inflammation leading to fibrosis is similar. In this case, just the etiology is known.

The collagen vascular diseases—systemic lupus erythematosus, rheumatoid arthritis, scleroderma, polymyositis/dermatomyositis, mixed connective tissue disease, ankylosing spondylitis, relapsing polychondritis, and Sjögren's syndrome—can each cause inflammation and injury of the lung parenchyma, central airways, pulmonary vasculature, and pleura.

Miliary rheumatoid nodules

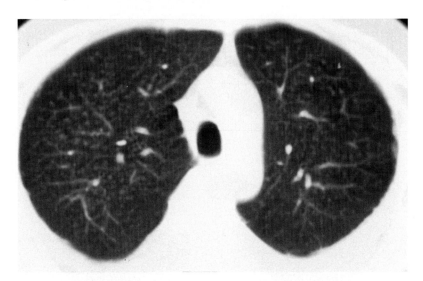

FIGURE 8-19

CT scan shows a diffuse miliary nodular infiltrate throughout both lungs. This is a very unusual early manifestation of rheumatoid lung. The term rheumatoid lung disease encompasses a broad spectrum of morphologic changes that carry significantly different prognoses. Differential diagnostic considerations include miliary granulomatous infection, hematogenous metastases, and lymphoma.

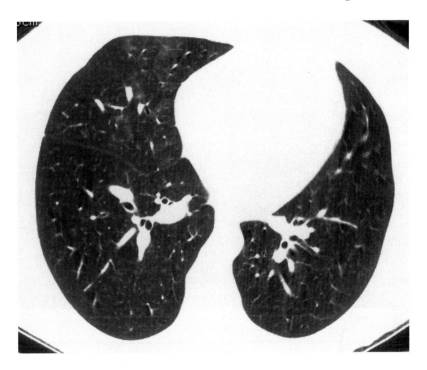

FIGURE 8-20

HRCT scan in a patient with rheumatoid arthritis shows patchy ground-glass opacities in the right middle lobe. A wide variety of pulmonary histopathologic features are seen in rheumatoid arthritis, many of which can cause ground-glass opacities: pulmonary rheumatoid nodules, usual interstitial pneumonia, bronchiolitis obliterans with patchy organizing pneumonia, lymphoid hyperplasia, and cellular interstitial infiltrates.[6]

Polymyositis

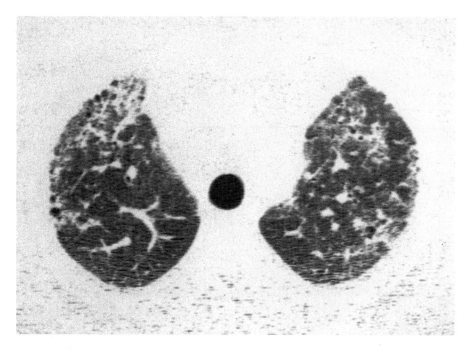

FIGURE 8-21

HRCT scan from this patient with polymyositis shows typical features of usual interstitial pneumonia. As in other collagen vascular diseases, nonspecific histologic patterns are found on lung biopsy: bronchiolitis obliterans organizing pneumonia (BOOP), usual interstitial pneumonia, and diffuse alveolar damage. Patients with BOOP have a more favorable prognosis than patients with usual interstitial pneumonia or diffuse alveolar damage.[7]

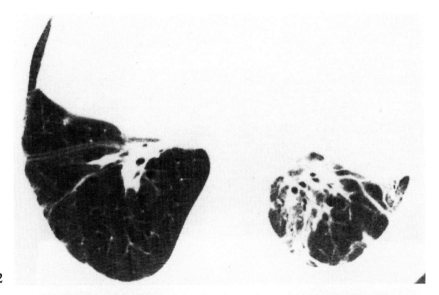

Figure 8-22

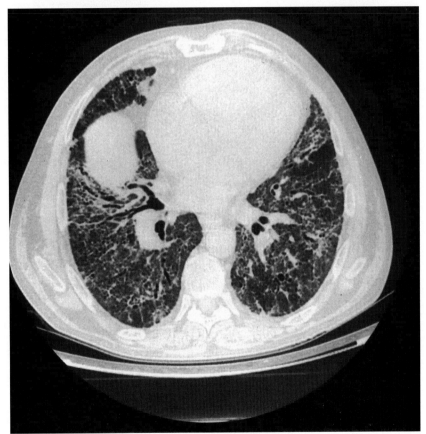

Figure 8-23

FIGURES 8-22 and 8-23

HRCT scans from two patients with dermatomyositis show a reticular infiltrative process in the lung bases with architectural distortion, including traction bronchiectasis. The upper lungs were spared. The findings are compatible with the pathologic diagnosis of usual interstitial pneumonia associated with dermatomyositis.

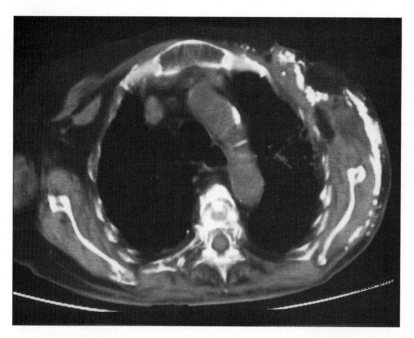

FIGURE 8-24

CT scan from this patient with dermatomyositis shows platelike calcification of some of the musculature and subcutaneous fat in the left hemithorax. Soft tissue calcifications can be seen in patients with dermatomyositis, chronic renal failure, myositis ossificans, and other conditions.

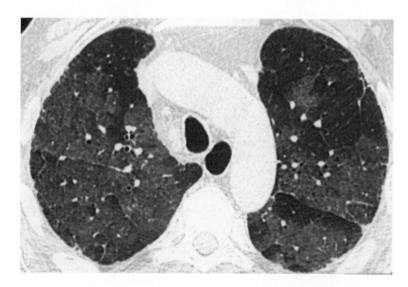

FIGURE 8-25

HRCT scan from this patient with dermatomyositis shows bilateral confluent regions of ground-glass opacity. Ground-glass opacity on HRCT is a nonspecific finding and can be seen in desquamative interstitial pneumonia, hypersensitivity pneumonitis, and cardiogenic and noncardiogenic edema, to name just a few etiologies. If there is no evidence of architectural distortion or traction bronchiectasis, ground-glass opacity is generally indicative of reversible disease.

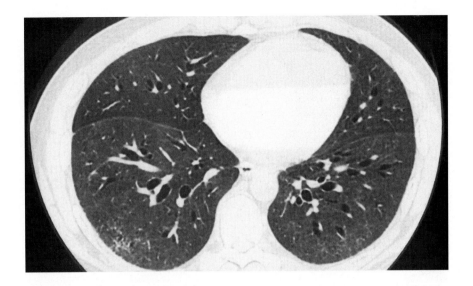

FIGURE 8-26

HRCT scan from a patient with scleroderma shows diffuse ground-glass opacity throughout the lung bases. Note marked dilatation of the basilar bronchi owing to traction. In this case, the ground-glass opacity should be caused by fibrosis because there is architectural distortion; it is probably not reversible. This patient's middle and upper lungs were uninvolved according to HRCT examination.

Diffuse pulmonary hemorrhage

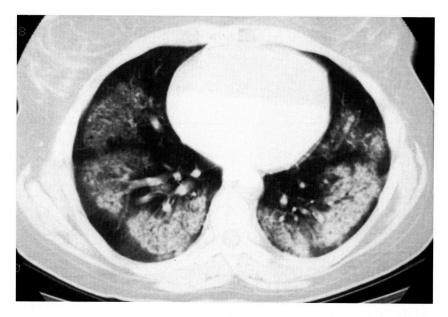

FIGURE 8-27

CT scan from a patient with systemic lupus erythematosus shows bilateral basilar regions of consolidation caused by diffuse pulmonary hemorrhage from pulmonary capillaritis. These were acute findings and cleared significantly within several days.

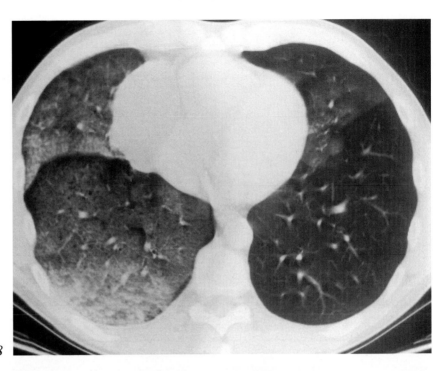

Figure 8-28

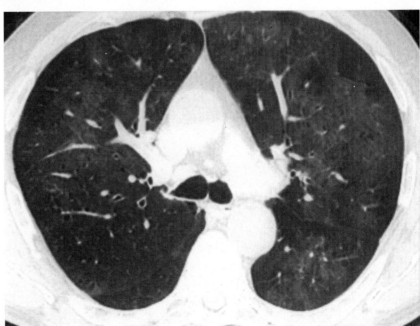

Figure 8-29

FIGURES 8-28 and 8-29

HRCT scans from two patients with cryptogenic intra-alveolar hemorrhage show a diffuse ground-glass pattern. This is a nonspecific pattern and may resemble pneumonia or other inflammatory processes.

Amiodarone toxicity

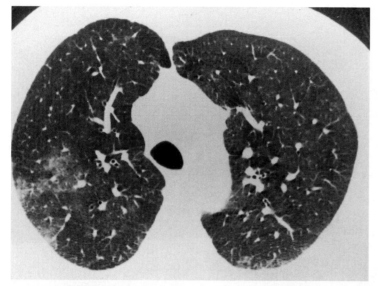

Figure 8-30

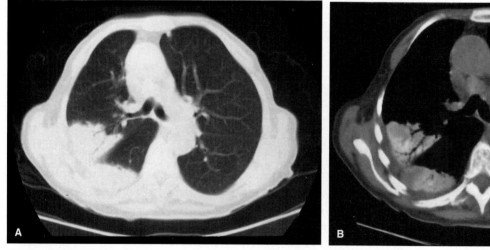

Figure 8-31

FIGURES 8-30 and 8-31

CT scans from two patients with amiodarone pulmonary toxicity. In Figure 8-30 note patchy areas of ground-glass opacification distributed diffusely throughout both lungs. In the patient in Figure 8-31, there are airless regions in the posterior segment of the right upper lobe and superior segment of the right lower lobe. These consolidated regions show considerable attenuation or "enhancement" in the absence of administration of any intravenous contrast material.

Amiodarone is an antiarrhythmic agent that contains iodine. Pulmonary toxicity can occur and probably reflects direct toxic effects as well as indirect inflammatory and immunologic processes.[8] In other patients with amiodarone toxicity, CT has demonstrated intralobular septal thickening and visceral pleural thickening.[9]

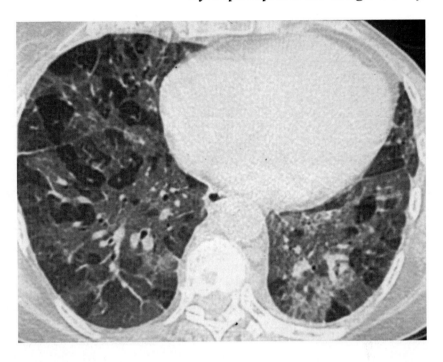

FIGURE 8-32

HRCT scan from a patient with cyclophosphamide drug toxicity shows ground-glass opacities, predominantly at the lung bases.

Cyclophosphamide, like numerous antineoplastic drugs, has pulmonary toxic side effects. Mechanisms include direct pulmonary toxicity and indirect effects through inflammatory reactions. Clinical features are similar for most agents—chronic pneumonitis and fibrosis. The number of drugs known or suspected of causing pulmonary toxicity is steadily increasing and includes bleomycin, procainamide, nitrofurantoin, cyclophosphamide, penicillamine, busulfan, carmustine, amiodarone, mitomycin, and methotrexate, among others.

HRCT can show a variety of findings in patients with pulmonary drug toxicity. They include (1) fibrosis with or without air space consolidation, (2) ground-glass opacities, (3) widespread bilateral air space consolidation, and (4) bronchial wall thickening with distal areas of decreased lung attenuation reflecting air trapping in obliterative bronchiolitis.[10]

Bleomycin toxicity

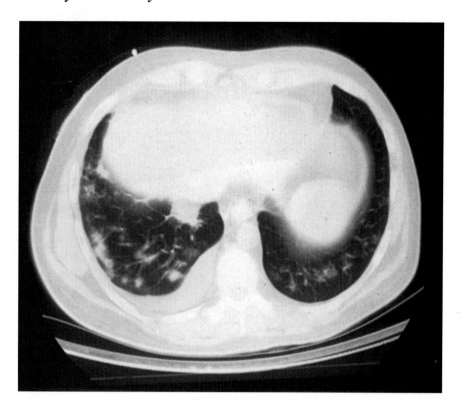

FIGURE 8-33

CT scan from a patient with bleomycin toxicity shows nodular opacities in the lung bases. These nodules may simulate pulmonary hematogenous metastases, causing considerable clinical concern.

There is a spectrum of bleomycin lung toxic effects that can range from an acute hypersensitivity reaction, to lung nodules, to diffuse alveolar damage leading to irreversible lung fibrosis.

REFERENCES

1. Remy-Jardin M, Giraud F, Remy J, Copin MC, Gosselin B, Duhamel A. Importance of ground-glass attenuation in chronic diffuse infiltrative lung disease: Pathologic-CT correlation. Radiology 1993; 189:693–698

2. Aquino SL, Webb WR, Zaloudek CJ, Stern EJ. Lung cysts associated with honeycombing: Change in size on expiratory CT scans. AJR 1994; 162:583–584

3. Daroca PJJ, George WJ. Giant cell interstitial pneumonia. South Med J 1991; 84: 257–263

4. Vedal S, Welsh EV, Miller RR, Müller NL. Desquamative interstitial pneumonia. Computed tomographic findings before and after treatment with corticosteroids. Chest 1988; 93:215–217

5. Schmid ZA, Bernheim R, Medici TC. Idiopathic lung fibrosis. Schweiz Med Wochenschr 1988; 118:979–985

6. Yousem SA, Colby TV, Carrington CB. Lung biopsy in rheumatoid arthritis. Am Rev Respir Dis 1985; 131:770–777

7. Tazelaar HD, Viggiano RW, Pickersgill J, Colby TV. Interstitial lung disease in polymyositis and dermatomyositis. Clinical features and prognosis as correlated with histologic findings. Am Rev Respir Dis 1990; 141:727–733

8. Martin WJ, Rosenow EC. Amiodarone pulmonary toxicity. Recognition and pathogenesis (Part 2). Chest 1988; 93:1242–1248

9. Ren H, Kuhlman JE, Hruban RH, Fishman EK, Wheeler PS, Hutchins GM. CT-pathology correlation of amiodarone lung. J Comput Assist Tomogr 1990; 14:760–765

10. Padley SP, Adler B, Hansell DM, Müller NL. High-resolution computed tomography of drug-induced lung disease. Clin Radiol 1992; 46:232–236

High-Resolution CT of the Chest: Comprehensive Atlas
by Eric J. Stern and Stephen J. Swensen,
Lippincott–Raven Publishers, Philadelphia © 1996.

Asbestos-Related Diseases
9

Asbestosis
Asymmetric asbestosis
Thick calcified pleural plaques
Thin calcified pleural plaques
Thin noncalcified pleural plaques
Diffuse pleural thickening
Rounded atelectasis

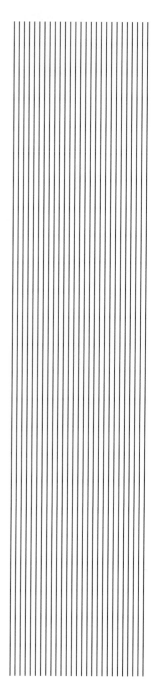

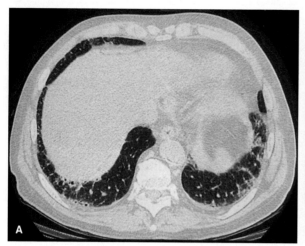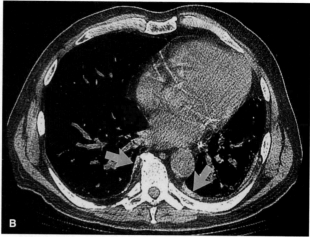

FIGURE 9-1

HRCT scans from a patient with lung fibrosis and asbestos exposure show the typical findings of usual interstitial pneumonia, in this case, asbestosis. These include predominantly basilar subpleural reticular infiltrative and fibrotic processes.

Early changes are often most evident in the dorsum of the lung, in which case images in the prone position are useful to differentiate true infiltrative lung disease from the gravity-dependent opacity that may be present (Figs. 14-6 through 14-8). Many patients with asbestosis have pleural plaques that indicate a significant exposure to asbestos (*arrows*). There also may be honeycombing, although not in this case.

The HRCT scan findings that correlate with clinical and occupational features of asbestosis include parenchymal bands, thickened interlobular septa, thickened intralobular core structures, subpleural lines, nondependent subpleural lung opacity, ground-glass lung opacities, traction bronchiectasis, and honeycombing (in advanced cases).[1,2]

Pathologically, thickened intralobular core structures are caused by peribronchiolar fibrosis. Thickened interlobular septa result from either interlobular fibrotic thickening or edema. The confluence of subpleural peribronchiolar fibrosis creates the subpleural curvilinear line. Subpleural fibrosis can extend proximally along the bronchovascular bundle to form parenchymal bands. Ground-glass opacities arise from mild alveolar wall and interlobular septal thickening produced by fibrosis or edema that is beyond the limits of resolution of HRCT, causing a generalized increase in background density.[3]

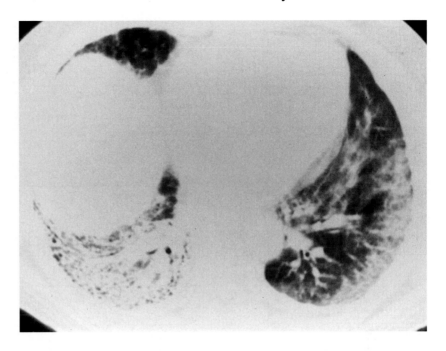

FIGURE 9-2

HRCT scan shows asymmetric pulmonary fibrosis with honeycombing involving predominantly the right lower lobe with only mild fibrotic changes noted in the left lower lobe. This is an unusual pattern of asbestosis.

Thick calcified pleural plaques

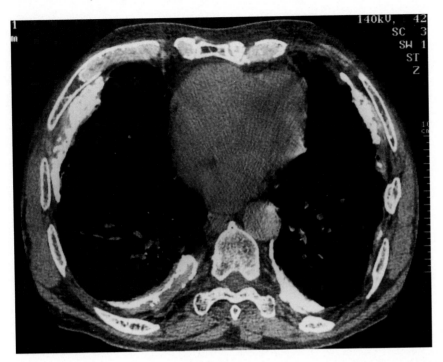

FIGURE 9-3

HRCT scan shows bilateral extensive thick calcified pleural plaques in this patient with occupational exposure to asbestos. The plaques are in typical locations: posterior/paravertebral and anterolateral pleural surfaces. Extensive calcified diaphragmatic plaques were also present (not shown). Pleural plaques can be caused by asbestos exposure; these plaques usually involve the parietal pleura. There is a 50% chance of forming pleural plaques about 30 years from the time of first exposure to asbestos fibers. Visceral pleural thickening, best seen in the pleural fissures, is common in asbestos exposure and is also related to the years since first asbestos exposure. Pleural plaques are not associated with clinically significant reductions in pulmonary function, and pleural plaques are not predictive of asbestosis. There are five asbestos-related pleural diseases: mesothelioma and four benign pleural reactions—pleural effusions, calcified or noncalcified pleural plaques, diffuse pleural thickening, and rounded atelectasis.

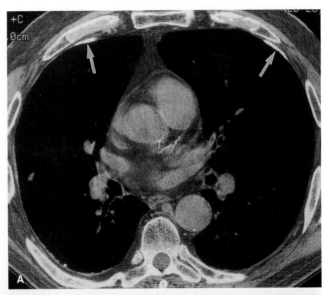

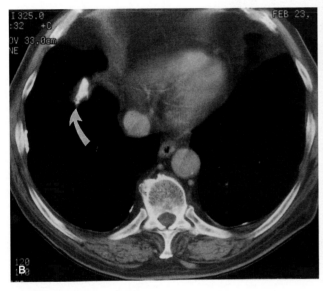

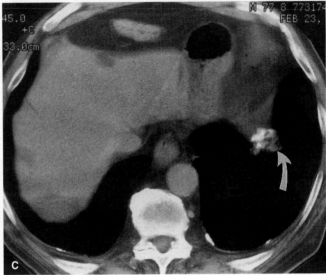

FIGURE 9-4

HRCT scans show bilateral, thin, partially calcified pleural plaques in typical locations (*arrows*) in this patient with occupational exposure to asbestos. Note the plaques on top of each hemidiaphragm (*curved arrows*).

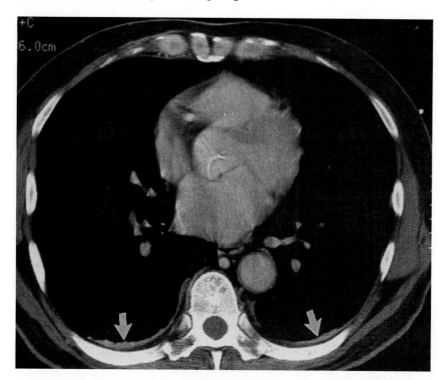

FIGURE 9-5

HRCT scan from this patient with occupational exposure to asbestos shows bilateral, thin, noncalcified pleural plaques (*arrows*).

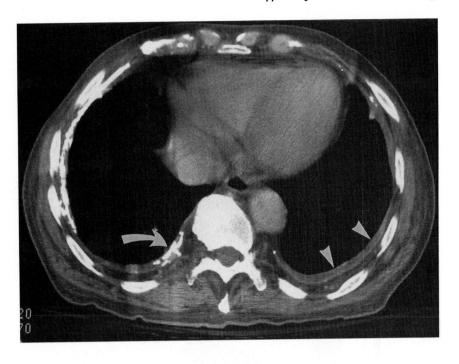

FIGURE 9-6

HRCT scan shows extensive pleural disease in this patient with occupational expo-sure to asbestos. In the right hemithorax is a large calcified pleural plaque (*curved arrow*). In the left hemithorax, however, is an area of diffuse pleural thickening (*ar-rowheads*), a smooth, noninterrupted pleural opacity extending over at least one fourth of the chest wall. Diffuse pleural thickening is usually caused by the residua of a benign asbestos-related pleuritis with pleural effusion or confluent pleural plaques. Diffuse pleural thickening may be physiologically significant; it may cause restrictive pulmonary function. Associated pulmonary fibrosis is infrequent.[4]

Rounded atelectasis

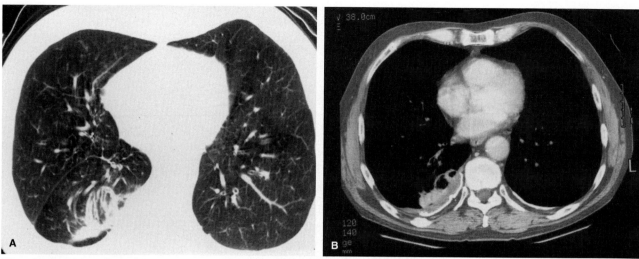

Figure 9-7

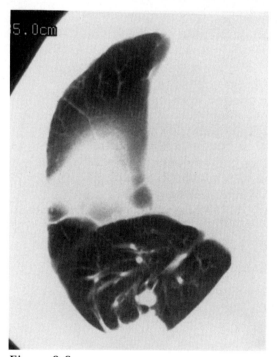

Figure 9-8

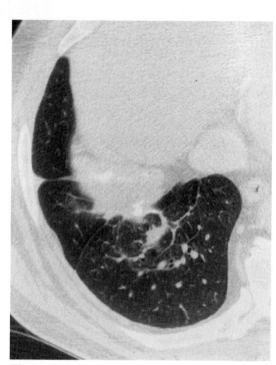

Figure 9-9

FIGURES 9-7, 9-8, and 9-9

HRCT scans from three different patients with rounded atelectasis show the typical rounded or wedge-shaped, pleural-based pulmonary opacity with vessels sweeping into the center. Asbestos-related rounded atelectasis is a nonmalignant radiographic consequence of asbestos exposure that can mimic lung cancer. It occurs in the lung periphery and is caused by pleural adhesions and fibrosis causing deformation of the lung. It can occur after any insult that causes pleural scarring, including surgery, trauma, or infection, as well as asbestos-related pleural disease.

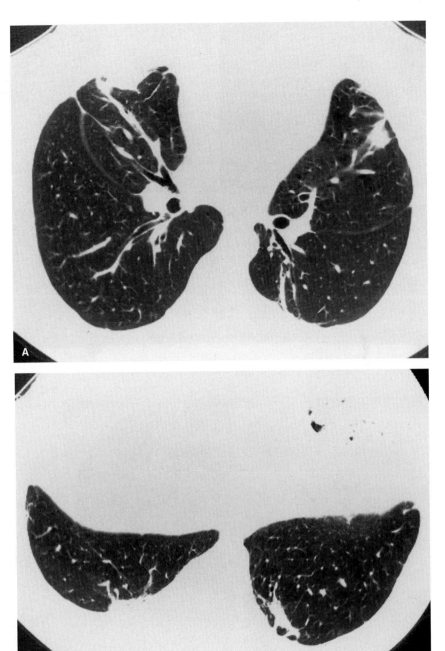

FIGURE 9-10

HRCT scans from this patient with occupational exposure to asbestos show four separate and distinct areas of rounded atelectasis, two anteriorly and two posteriorly. Rounded atelectasis is usually a solitary finding, although it may be multiple, as in this case, and can involve any lobe of the lung,[5] although the posterior lung bases are the most common sites.

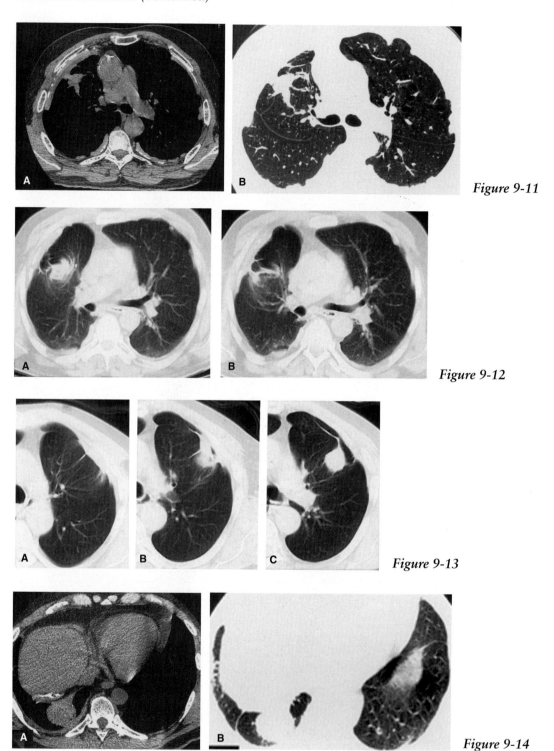

Figure 9-11

Figure 9-12

Figure 9-13

Figure 9-14

FIGURES 9-11, 9-12, 9-13, and 9-14

HRCT scans from four patients with rounded atelectasis all show a similarity to findings in patients with lung cancers. Note the contiguity of the "mass," with large, thick pleural plaques as a distinguishing, although not pathognomonic, feature. Sometimes it is impossible to radiologically distinguish rounded atelectasis from lung cancer.

REFERENCES

1. Gamsu G, Aberle DR, Lynch DA. Computed tomography in the diagnosis of asbestos-related thoracic disease. J Thorac Imaging 1989; 4:61–67

2. Lynch DA, Gamsu G, Aberle DR. Conventional and high resolution computed tomography in the diagnosis of asbestos-related diseases. Radiographics 1989; 9:523–551

3. Akira M, Yamamoto S, Yokoyama K, et al. Asbestosis: High-resolution CT-pathologic correlation. Radiology 1990; 176:389–394

4. McLoud TC, Woods BO, Carrington CB, Epler GR, Gaensler EA. Diffuse pleural thickening in an asbestos-exposed population: Prevalence and causes. AJR 1985; 144:9–18

5. Hillerdal G. Rounded atelectasis. Clinical experience with 74 patients. Chest 1989; 95:836–841

High-Resolution CT of the Chest: Comprehensive Atlas
by Eric J. Stern and Stephen J. Swensen,
Lippincott–Raven Publishers, Philadelphia © 1996.

Lung Masses
10

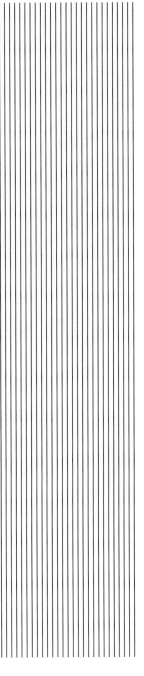

Bronchioloalveolar carcinoma

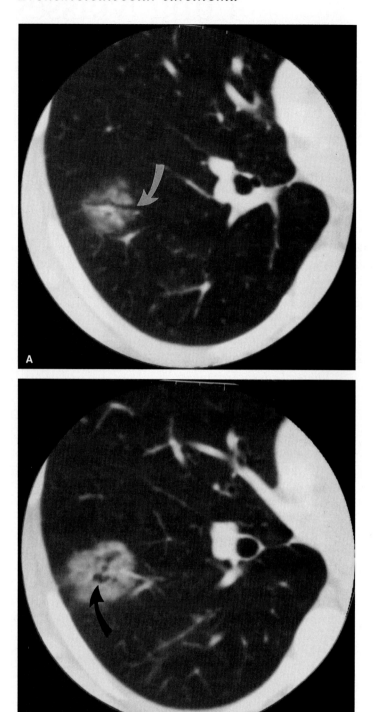

FIGURE 10-1

HRCT scans from this patient with bronchioloalveolar carcinoma show a 4 cm, masslike region of consolidation in the anterior basal segment of the right lower lobe. The mass contains air bronchograms (*arrows*), suggesting the neoplastic differential diagnosis of bronchioloalveolar carcinoma or lymphoma.

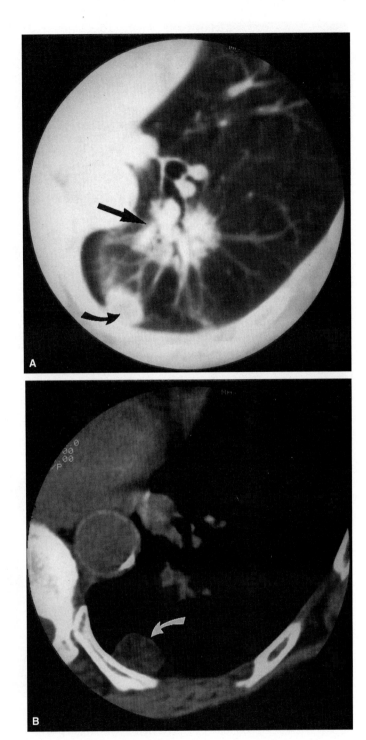

FIGURE 10-2

HRCT scan shows a 4 cm, masslike region of consolidation in the superior segment of the left lower lobe that contains air bronchograms (*straight arrow*) compatible with bronchioloalveolar carcinoma (A). There is a second 2.5 cm mass (*curved arrow*) that soft-tissue windows show contains fat attenuation (B) compatible with a pulmonary hamartoma.

Figure 10-3

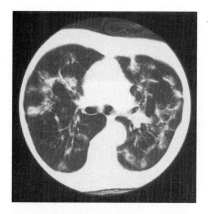

Figure 10-4

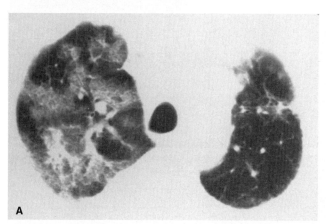

A

Upper lung zone

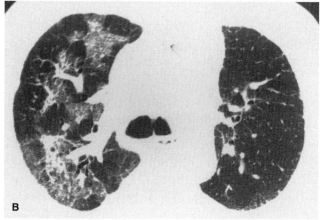

B

Middle lung zone

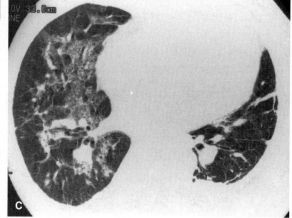

C

Lower lung zone

FIGURES 10-3 and 10-4

HRCT scans from two patients with multifocal bronchioloalveolar carcinoma show ill-defined patchy areas of attenuation, some with a ground-glass attenuation, others more consolidated. This malignancy can be bilateral (Fig. 10-3) or asymmetric (Fig. 10-4). Approximately 15% to 25% of bronchioloalveolar carcinomas are disseminated at time of presentation; when disseminated, as above, the tumor is unresectable and the prognosis is very poor.

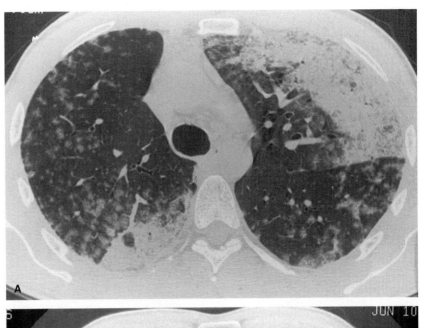

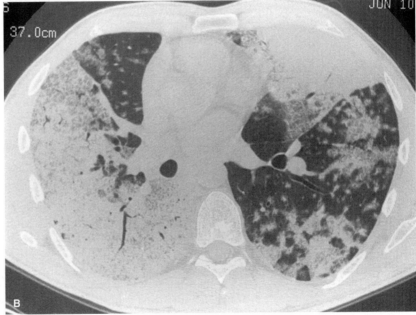

FIGURE 10-5

HRCT scans from a patient with multifocal bronchioloalveolar carcinoma show multifocal regions of consolidated parenchyma with air bronchograms as well as multiple ill-defined small rounded opacities suggesting endobronchial dissemination. These features are nonspecific and may represent any air space filling process such as pneumonia or pulmonary hemorrhage. The clinical context of nonresolving or progressive infiltrates in a patient lacking signs and symptoms of an infection is very important in suggesting the diagnosis of bronchioloalveolar carcinoma.

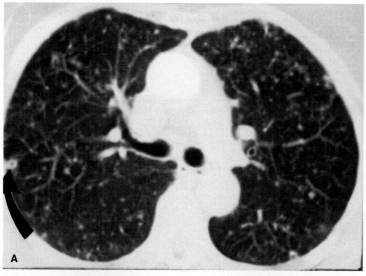

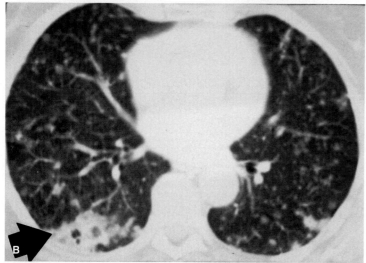

FIGURE 10-6

CT scans from a patient with multifocal bronchioloalveolar carcinoma show a diffuse, small nodular infiltrative process throughout both lungs with no basilar, apical, central, or peripheral predominance. Some of the nodules are cavitated (*curved arrow*). There is a focal region of masslike consolidation in the posterior and lateral basal segments of the right lower lobe (*arrow*). Approximately 15% to 25% of bronchioloalveolar carcinoma cases are disseminated at the time of presentation, as in this case.

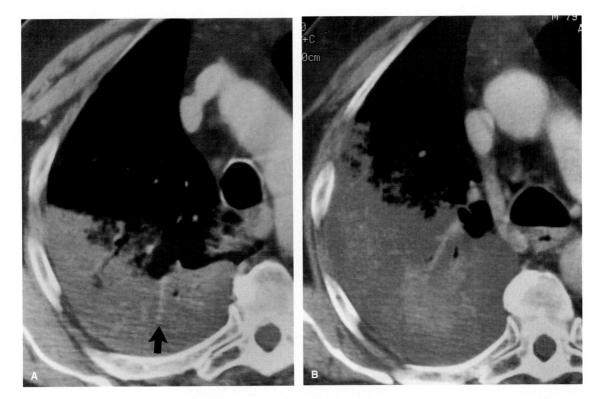

FIGURE 10-7

CT scans from this patient with bronchioloalveolar carcinoma show an area of dense consolidation in the right lower lobe. Note the enhancing pulmonary vessels (*arrow*) within the low density (water density) area of attenuation (the CT angiogram sign)—a drowned-lung appearance. Tumor or the excessive mucus production seen with bronchioloalveolar carcinoma gives this appearance, but is nonspecific and may be seen in other processes that obstruct the airways, causing mucus to build up behind the obstruction.

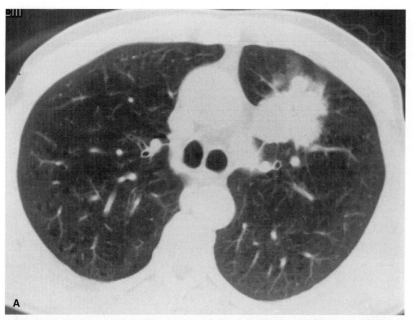

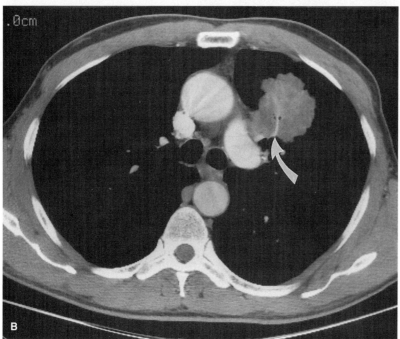

FIGURE 10-8

CT scan from this patient with a left upper lobe adenocarcinoma (A) shows enhancing pulmonary vessels (*arrow*) (B) within the low density (water) mass (the CT angiogram sign). This is a nonspecific sign that is suggestive of malignancy but can be seen in other etiologies of lung consolidation.

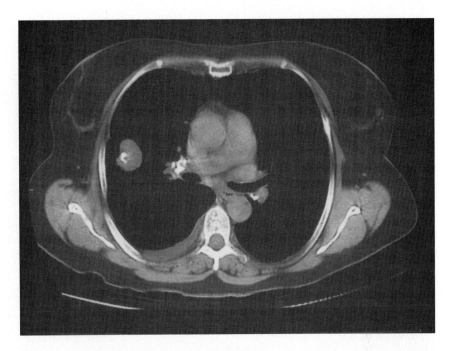

FIGURE 10-9

CT scan shows a 2.5 cm nodule in the right upper lobe that contains *eccentric* calcification and calcified hilar lymph nodes. Because eccentric calcification is an indeterminate indicator of a benign process, the lung nodule was resected and proved to be an adenocarcinoma. The calcification was a granuloma that had been engulfed by the bronchogenic carcinoma. This lung cancer may have developed as a "scar carcinoma." In order to be considered benign, calcification must be central, diffuse, laminated, or chondroid ("popcorn").

Carcinoma with dystrophic calcification

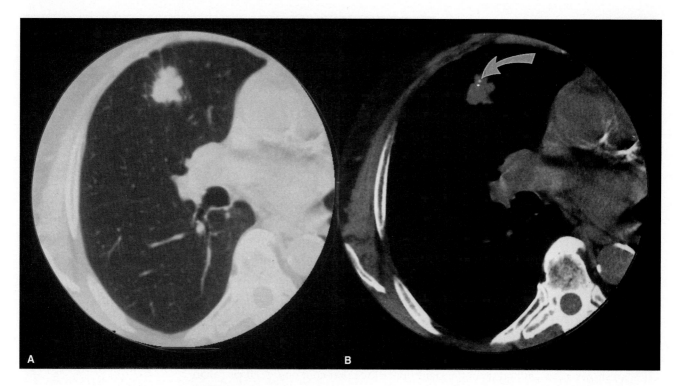

FIGURE 10-10

HRCT scans show a small amount of eccentric calcification (*arrow*) in this lobulated, spiculated, 3 cm mass in the anterior segment of the right upper lobe. This eccentric calcification is not indicative of a benign process. After surgical resection, this was shown to be a squamous cell carcinoma with dystrophic calcification.

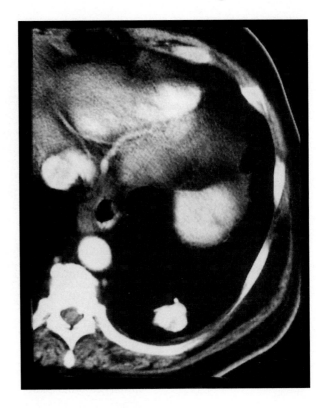

FIGURE 10-11

Contrast-enhanced CT scan shows a 2.5 cm very homogeneously dense nodule in the left lower lobe. It appears to be "calcified" in a benign pattern. Thin sections through this nodule 5 minutes after this image was obtained showed no evidence of calcification. The apparent calcification was caused by intense enhancement of this vascular primary adenocarcinoma of the lung. This is a pitfall to bear in mind, particularly with fast CT scanners. Lung nodule enhancement can be an indication of malignancy.[1]

Adenocarcinoma with hematogenous metastases

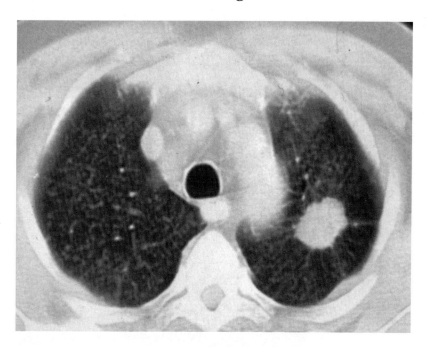

FIGURE 10-12

CT scan from a patient with adenocarcinoma of the left upper lobe shows a diffuse miliary nodular pattern caused by hematogenous metastases from the primary malignancy. This miliary nodular pattern is nonspecific and can be seen with other malignant or infectious processes.

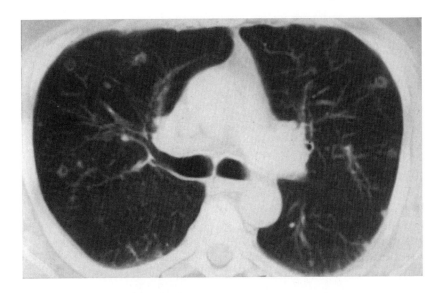

FIGURE 10-13

CT scan from a patient with metastatic pancreatic adenocarcinoma shows multiple bilateral small pulmonary nodules, many of which are cavitated. Other differential diagnostic possibilities would include disseminated granulomatous infection, lymphoproliferative disorder, and less commonly Wegener's granulomatosis.

Non-Hodgkin's lymphoma

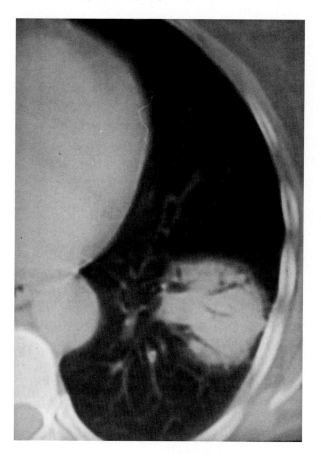

FIGURE 10-14

CT scan from a patient with primary non-Hodgkin's lymphoma of the lung shows a 4 cm, masslike region of consolidation in the left lower lobe. Note the air bronchograms that form within this soft tumor. Round pneumonia and bronchioloalveolar carcinoma can have a similar appearance.

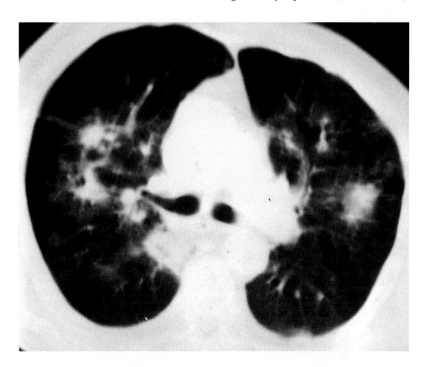

FIGURE 10-15

CT scan from a patient with primary non-Hodgkin's lymphoma of the lung shows patchy bilateral predominantly perihilar regions of consolidation and interstitial infiltrate. There is mediastinal and hilar lymphadenopathy. Differential diagnostic considerations include sarcoidosis, bronchioloalveolar carcinoma, and granulomatous infection.

Cavitary squamous cell carcinoma

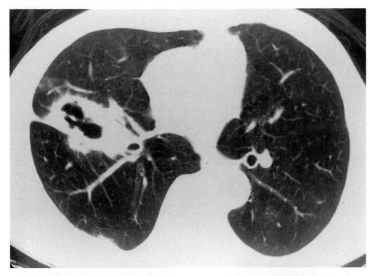

Figure 10-16

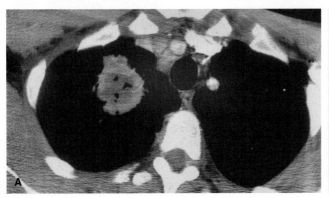

Figure 10-17

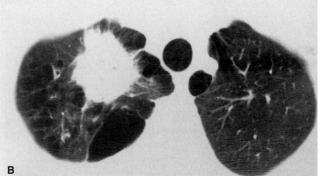

FIGURES 10-16 and 10-17

CT scans from two patients with squamous cell carcinoma of the lung show large lung masses with central necrosis and cavitation. Squamous cell carcinomas, closely associated with cigarette smoking, are the most common lung malignancies to cavitate, especially with increasing size.

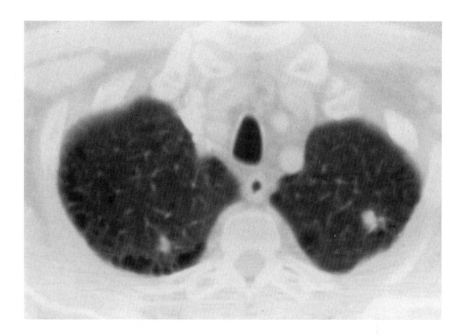

FIGURE 10-18

CT scan shows bilateral apical spiculated lung masses surgically proved to be synchronous lung cancers. The incidence of detection of multiple primary bronchogenic carcinomas has increased with the advent of CT; incidence of detection is generally considered to be 1% of lung cancers. Most patients are heavy smokers. Multiple primary bronchogenic carcinomas may be bilateral, synchronous, or metachronous.[2] Incidental note is made of paraseptal emphysema (see Figs. 7-13 through 7-16).

Pulmonary hamartoma

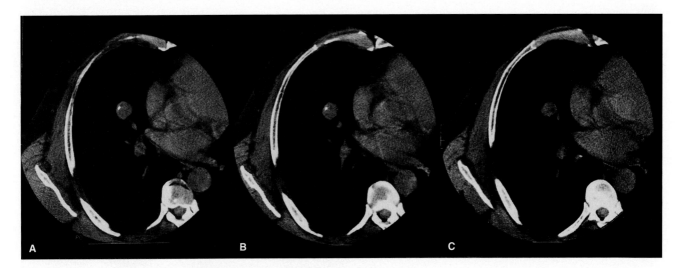

FIGURE 10-19

HRCT scans show a 2 cm smoothly marginated lung nodule in the middle lobe containing focal areas of fat and eccentric chondroid calcification. Findings are characteristic of pulmonary hamartoma, confirmed at surgery.

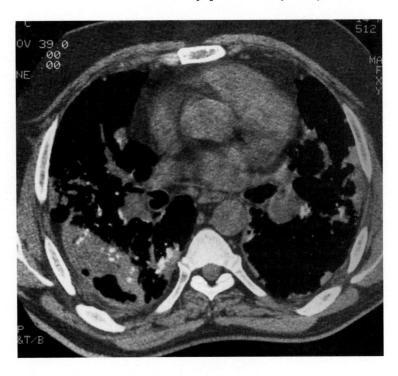

FIGURE 10-20

HRCT scan through the midlung in this patient with primary pulmonary amyloidosis shows confluent subpleural opacities containing several calcific foci.

Primary pulmonary amyloidosis is a rare disease that occurs in three forms: (1) tracheobronchial, (2) nodular parenchymal, and (3) the least common but most clinically significant, diffuse parenchymal or alveolar septal amyloidosis, as in this case. In the alveolar septal form, amyloid deposition in the lung is often widespread, involving small blood vessels and the parenchymal interstitium, and multifocal small nodules of amyloid may be present. Patients with diffuse parenchymal amyloidosis are more likely to die of respiratory failure than are patients with the two other forms of the disease. Radiologically, alveolar septal amyloidosis appears as nonspecific diffuse interstitial or alveolar opacities which, once established, change very little over time. The abnormal areas can calcify or, rarely, show frank ossification. Calcification of small interstitial nodules may also be seen in silicosis and coal-worker's pneumoconiosis.

Carcinoid tumor

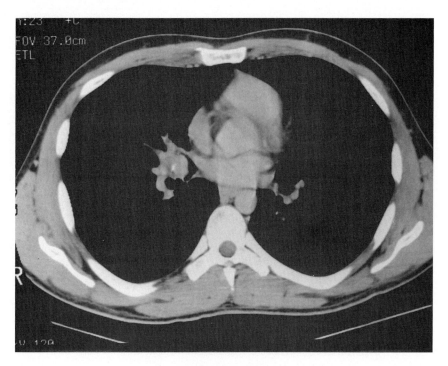

FIGURE 10-21

CT scan through the right hilum shows a 2 cm mass with central calcification, in this case, a carcinoid tumor. CT detection of calcification within carcinoid tumors is not uncommon, seen in approximately 40% of central carcinoid tumors in one series.[3] Ossification by one of the bioactive secretions of the tumor is induced in the surrounding bronchial cartilage. This explains two features: (1) the chunky nature of the "calcifications" and (2) the predominance of this finding in central carcinoid tumors versus the relative lack of calcification in peripheral carcinoid tumors, where the bronchial cartilage is not present.[3]

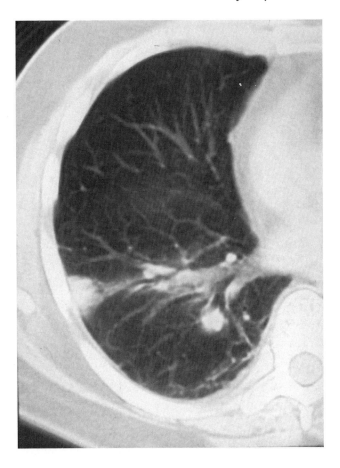

FIGURE 10-22

CT scan shows a 2 cm, wedge-shaped lung lesion abutting the pleura laterally. A bronchus and artery extend into the apex of this nodule. Although it is nonspecific, this appearance is typical of a pulmonary infarction.

Bronchocele

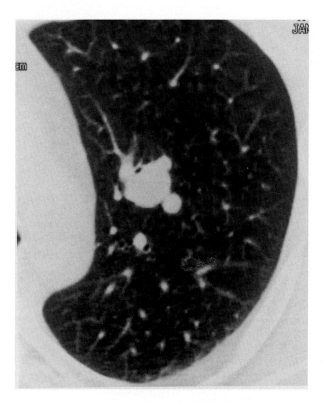

FIGURE 10-23

HRCT scan shows a rounded mass in the left upper lobe, closely associated with the bronchovascular bundle of the anterior segment. Contiguous scans showed this "mass" to be tubular, representing a mucus-filled bronchocele distal to an atretic airway of bronchial atresia. Expiratory CT scans (not shown) demonstrated air trapping in the anterior segmental bronchus distribution.

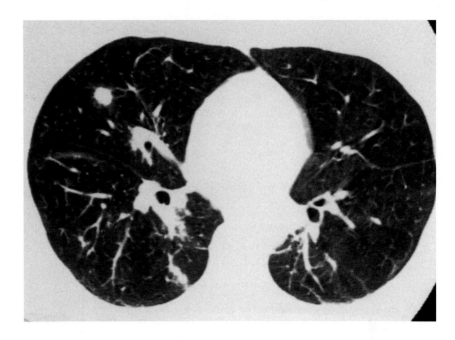

FIGURE 10-24

CT scan from this patient with Wegener's granulomatosis shows multiple pulmonary nodules with irregular margins.

Wegener's granulomatosis is characterized on CT scans as multiple nodules or masses with irregular margins, often with cavitation, and pleural-based pulmonary consolidations resembling pulmonary infarcts. Angiocentric forms of granulomatous vasculitis of the lung, as opposed to bronchocentric granulomatosis, include Wegener's granulomatosis, allergic angiitis and Churg-Strauss granulomatosis, lymphomatoid granulomatosis, and necrotizing sarcoid granulomatosis. Wegener's granulomatosis is a well-defined syndrome characterized by necrotizing granulomatous vasculitis of the upper (see Figs. 3-12 and 3-13) and lower respiratory tracts, segmental necrotizing glomerulonephritis, and systemic small vessel vasculitis. In Wegener's granulomatosis, improvement occasionally occurs in one area while disease progresses elsewhere in the lung.

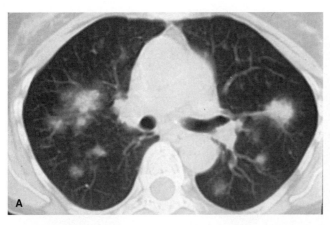
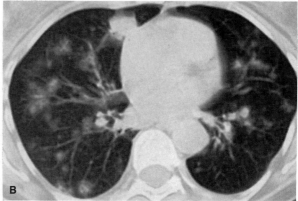

FIGURE 10-25

CT scans from this patient with Wegener's granulomatosis show multiple, bilateral, poorly circumscribed lung nodules and masses. Differential diagnostic considerations include bronchioloalveolar carcinoma, lymphoma, metastasis, disseminated granulomatous infection, sarcoidosis, and Wegener's granulomatosis.

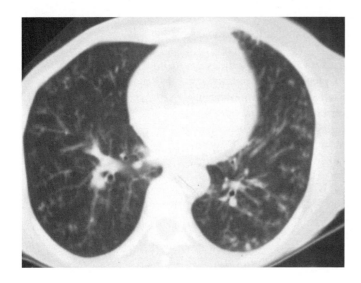

FIGURE 10-26

CT scan from a patient with Wegener's granulomatosis shows a more atypical pattern of diffuse bilateral nodular infiltrates. In this case, the distribution was uniform with no peripheral, central, basilar, or apical predominance.

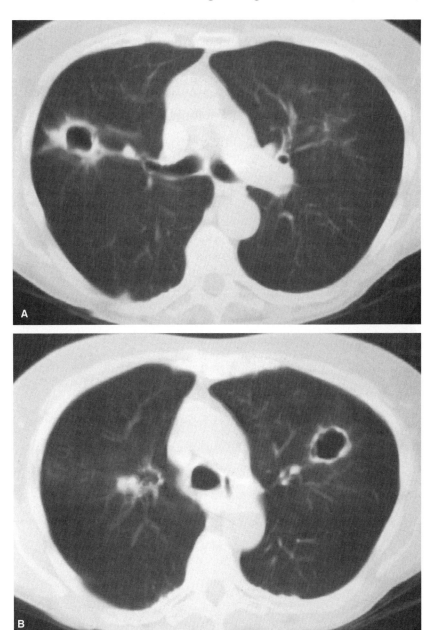

FIGURE 10-27

CT scans from a patient with Wegener's granulomatosis show cavitating nodules measuring approximately 3 cm in diameter in both upper lobes. The wall contour is irregular and mildly nodular. Lung masses of Wegener's granulomatosis often cavitate when their diameters are >2 cm.[4]

REFERENCES

1. Swensen SJ, Brown LR, Colby TV, Weaver AL. Pulmonary nodules: CT evaluation of enhancement with iodinated contrast material. Radiology 1995; 194:393–398

2. Kono M, Fujii M, Adachi S, Tanaka K, Shimizu T, Hirota S. Multiple primary lung cancers: Radiographic and bronchoscopic diagnosis. J Thorac Imaging 1993; 8:63–68

3. Zwiebel BR, Austin JH, Grimes MM. Bronchial carcinoid tumors: Assessment with CT of location and intratumoral calcification in 31 patients. Radiology 1991; 179:483–486

4. Weir IH, Müller NL, Chiles C, Godwin JD, Lee SH, Kullnig P. Wegener's granulomatosis: Findings from computed tomography of the chest in 10 patients. Can Assoc Radiol J 1992; 43:31–34

High-Resolution CT of the Chest: Comprehensive Atlas
by Eric J. Stern and Stephen J. Swensen,
Lippincott–Raven Publishers, Philadelphia © 1996.

Multiple Small Parenchymal Nodules

11

Sarcoidosis
Löfgren's syndrome
End-stage sarcoidosis
Berylliosis
Barium aspiration
Silicosis
Complicated silicosis
Alveolar microlithiasis
Metastatic calcification

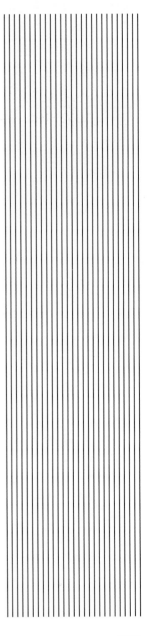

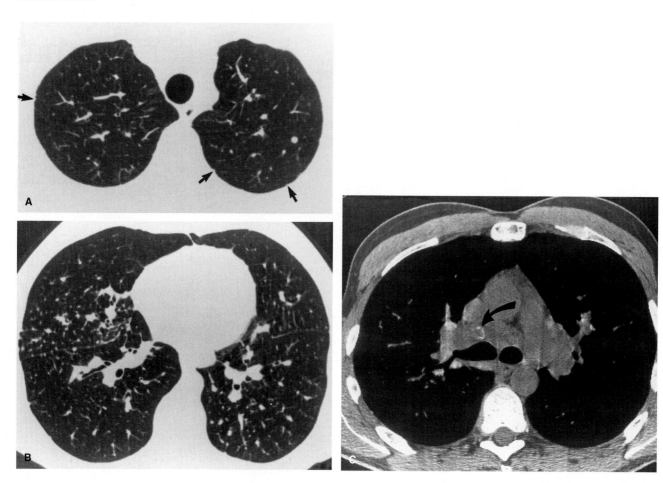

FIGURE 11-1

HRCT scans show a spectrum of findings in this patient with sarcoidosis. Note the small subpleural nodules in the upper lung zone (*arrows*), peribronchovascular nodular thickening in the middle zone, and adenopathy with eggshell hilar lymph node calcification (*curved arrow*).

Sarcoidosis is a systemic disorder characterized by widespread development of nonspecific, noncaseating granulomas. The etiology is unknown. Pulmonary disease associated with sarcoidosis may resolve spontaneously or progress to fibrosis (see Fig. 11-14). Because lymphadenopathy is the most common intrathoracic manifestation of sarcoidosis, the chest radiograph is abnormal in 90% to 95% of patients at some point, although 5% to 15% have a normal chest radiograph at initial presentation.

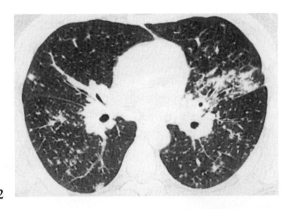

Figure 11-2

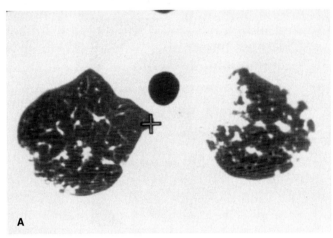

A

Upper lung zone

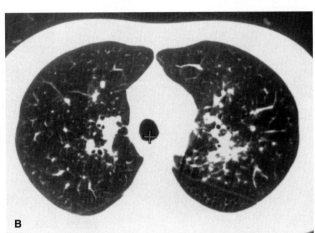

B

Middle lung zone

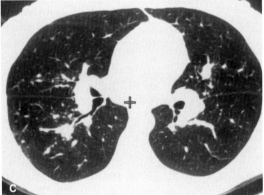

Figure 11-3

C

Lower lung zone

FIGURES 11-2 and 11-3

HRCT scans from two patients with sarcoidosis show relatively symmetric nodular infiltrates along peribronchovascular bundles. Subpleural nodules and hilar adenopathy are also noted.

In the lung, sarcoid granulomas are distributed primarily along the lymphatics, and therefore the peribronchovascular interstitial space, the interlobular septa, and the subpleural interstitial space are involved. Nodules represent coalescent granulomas, usually have irregular margins, and are typically 2 mm to 10 mm in diameter. Parenchymal opacities commonly involve the upper and middle lung zones but can also involve the lower lung zones.[1]

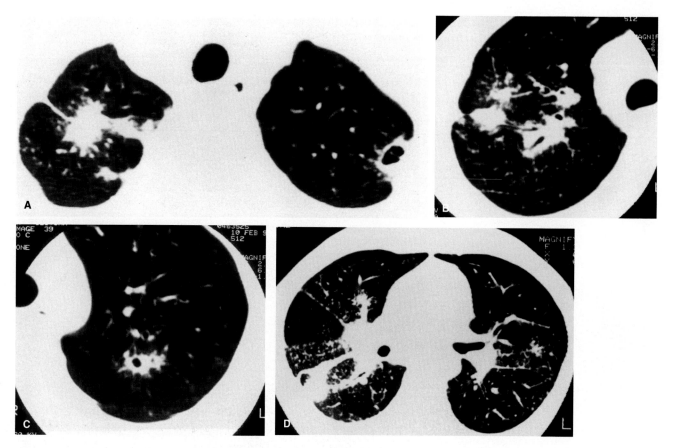

FIGURE 11-4

HRCT scans from this patient with sarcoidosis show many of the HRCT features of sarcoidosis and include nodules, masslike confluent nodules, fibrosis with lung architectural distortion and traction bronchiectasis, thickening of the pleural surfaces, ground-glass opacities, and air-filled cavities or cysts. In other words, sarcoidosis can have many different appearances, even within the same patient.

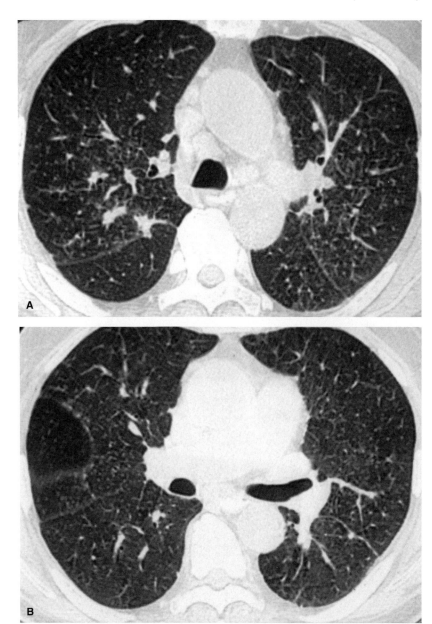

FIGURE 11-5

HRCT scans from a patient with sarcoidosis show a fine nodularity throughout the lung with minimal peribronchovascular thickening. There is a slight upper lobe predominance.

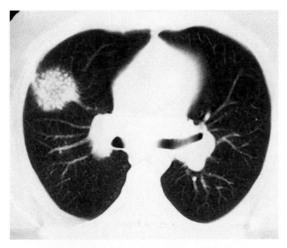

Figure 11-6

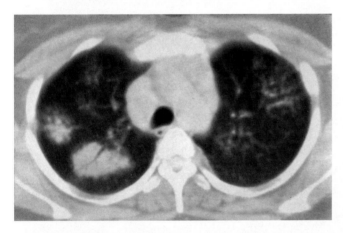

Figure 11-7

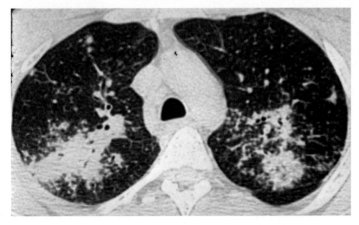

Figure 11-8

FIGURES 11-6, 11-7, and 11-8

HRCT scans from three patients with sarcoidosis show focal bilateral regions of masslike consolidation. This is an unusual manifestation of sarcoidosis, occurring in less than 5% of cases. Differential diagnostic considerations include lymphoma, Wegener's granulomatosis, bronchioloalveolar carcinoma, and bronchiolitis obliterans with organizing pneumonia. The clinical presentation can help distinguish these diseases.

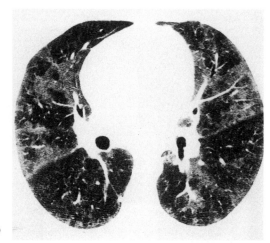

Figure 11-9

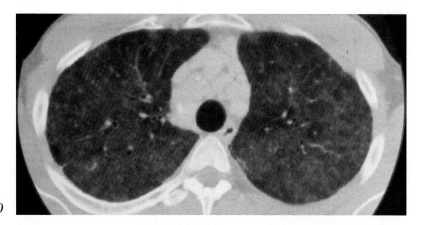

Figure 11-10

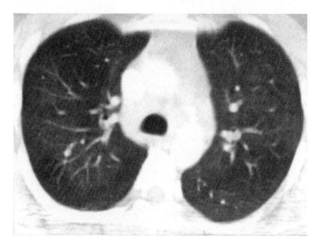

Figure 11-11

FIGURES 11-9, 11-10, and 11-11

HRCT scans from three patients with the ground-glass pattern of attenuation occasionally seen in sarcoidosis. The ground-glass attenuation is caused by alveolar granulomas and inflammation beyond the resolution limits of the CT scanner. Rarely, this appearance resembles that of alveolar proteinosis (see Fig. 2-22) or *Pneumocystic carinii* pneumonia (see Fig. 13-9).

Löfgren's syndrome

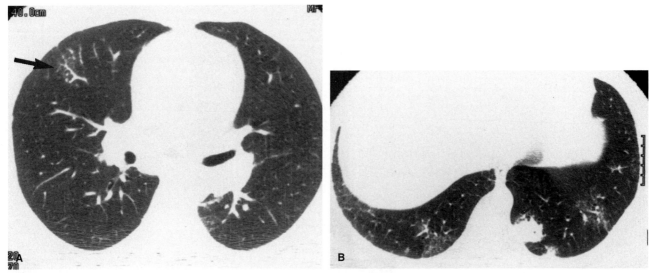

Figure 11-12

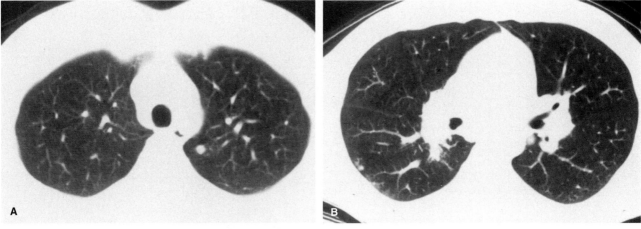

Figure 11-13

FIGURES 11-12 and 11-13

HRCT scans from two patients with a specific presentation of acute sarcoidosis called Löfgren's syndrome show subtle focal nodular infiltrates and ground-glass opacity (Fig. 11-12*B*) within the lungs. Note a "tree-in-bud" appearance (Fig. 11-12*A*) (*arrow*) similar to that seen in another active granulomatous process, tuberculosis (see Figs. 12-7 through 12-9). Patients with Löfgren's syndrome usually have fevers, skin lesions (usually erythema nodosum), arthralgias or polyarthralgias (usually of the foot, ankle, or other large joints), and hilar adenopathy. Lung parenchymal sarcoidosis is not generally appreciated on chest radiographs, as in these cases.

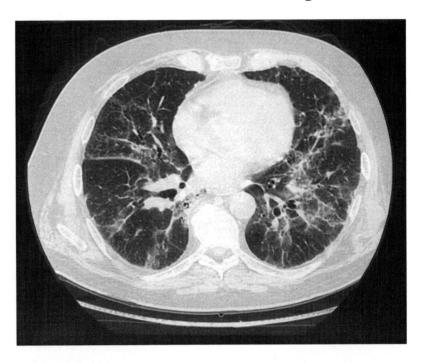

FIGURE 11-14

HRCT scan of a patient with end-stage sarcoidosis shows extensive lung fibrosis. The fibrotic infiltrative changes have resulted in architectural distortion, including traction bronchiectasis. There is still a relatively central distribution of the infiltrative process, which is characteristic of sarcoidosis.

Many of the parenchymal findings on HRCT scans can be considered representations of both reversible and irreversible disease. Nodules, irregularly marginated nodules, and alveolar or pseudoalveolar consolidation are inflammatory lesions that may be reversible with or without therapy, whereas septal thickening, nonseptal thickening, and lung distortion are usually fibrotic lesions that are irreversible.[2]

Sarcoidosis

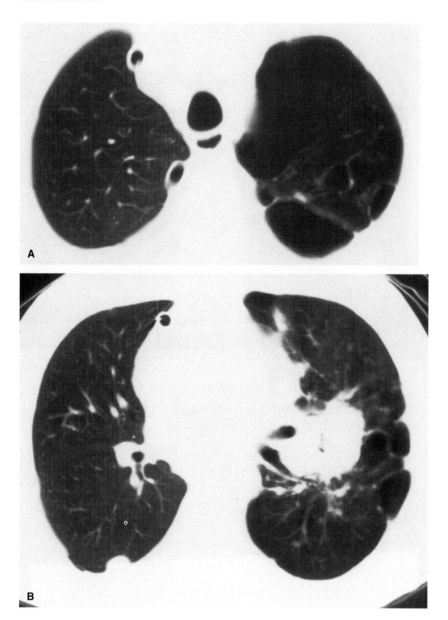

FIGURE 11-15

HRCT scans from this patient, performed after a right lung transplant for end-stage sarcoidosis, show both bullous disease and a conglomerate left perihilar mass in the native left lung. Sarcoidosis is one entity that causes upper lobe bullous/fibrobullous disease. Other entities include ankylosing spondylitis, progressive massive fibrosis of silicosis, and emphysema.

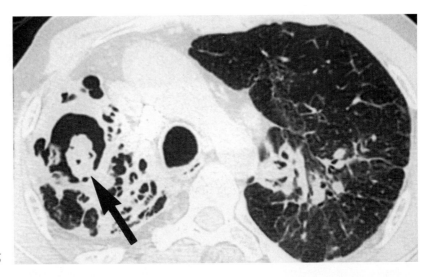

Figure 11-16

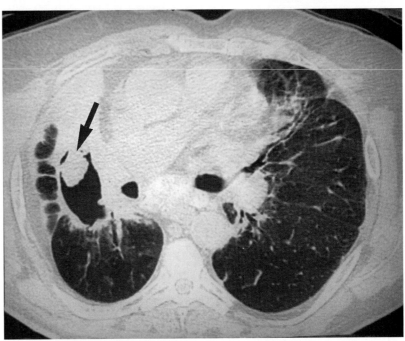

Figure 11-17

FIGURES 11-16 and 11-17

HRCT scans from two patients with cavitary/cystic sarcoidosis each show an aspergilloma in the right upper lobe cavities (*arrows*). There are extensive regions of traction bronchiectasis and architectural distortion, most marked in the right upper lobes in these patients with end-stage sarcoidosis. Associated pleural thickening is a common finding with an aspergilloma. Note that Figure 11-17 is an HRCT scan performed in the prone position and shows a mobile mycetoma within this pre-existing cavity.

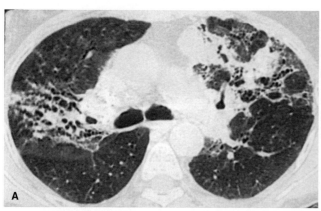
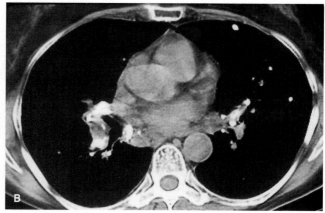

FIGURE 11-18

HRCT scan from a patient with berylliosis shows a bilateral, predominantly perihilar, fibrotic, infiltrative process with honeycombing and architectural distortion, including traction bronchiectasis. There are calcified nodules within the parenchymal process as well as calcified hilar and mediastinal nodes. Findings in berylliosis are indistinguishable from those of sarcoidosis both radiologically and pathologically. Berylliosis is a systemic disorder that results from exposure to beryllium. In its chronic form, it produces granulomatous and fibrotic disease in the lungs.

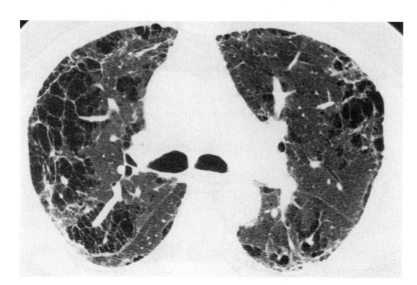

FIGURE 11-19

HRCT scan from this patient in the advanced stage of berylliosis shows a nonspecific, fibrotic, end-stage lung appearance.

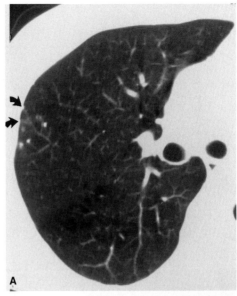

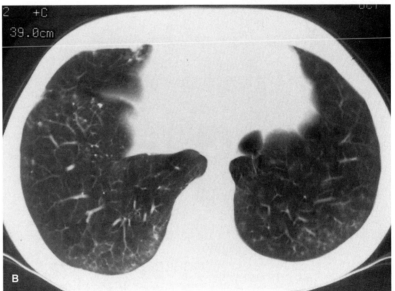

FIGURE 11-20

HRCT scans from a patient with barium aspiration show multiple, small, ill-defined nodular opacities distributed within one or two secondary pulmonary lobules (A), and a "tree-in-bud" appearance (*arrows*) similar to that of tuberculosis (see Figs. 12-7 through 12-9) and sarcoidosis (see Fig. 11-12), suggesting a granulomatous process. In (B), note similar scattered nodular opacities in a more typical distribution for aspiration.

Silicosis

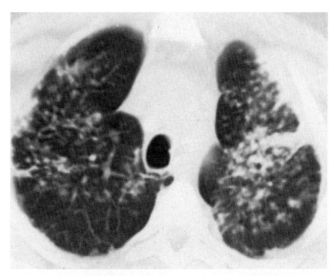

Figure 11-21

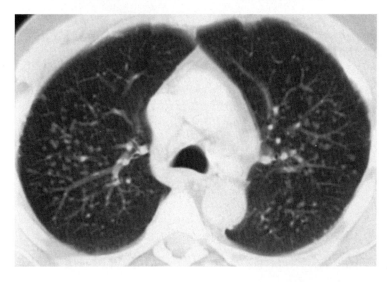

Figure 11-22

FIGURES 11-21 and 11-22

HRCT scans from two patients with silicosis show innumerable small rounded nodules in the lung parenchyma, predominantly in the upper lobes.

Silicosis is caused by inhalation of dust containing crystallized silicon dioxide. Coal-worker's pneumoconiosis results from inhalation of coal dust. The radiographic and CT abnormalities are the same for these two pneumoconioses and are characterized by the presence of small rounded nodules in the lung parenchyma, predominantly in the upper lobes, especially with milder disease. Nodules are typically centrilobular or subpleural in location, rarely calcified, sharply circumscribed, and usually measure 2 to 5 mm in diameter, although they may be up to 10 mm in diameter. Eggshell calcification may occur in mediastinal or hilar lymph nodes. These pneumoconioses can progress and be complicated by the development of large massive areas of fibrosis in the upper lung zones. Dyspnea in these patients is usually caused by superimposed emphysema rather than the silicotic nodules; the emphysema is easily detected on HRCT.[3]

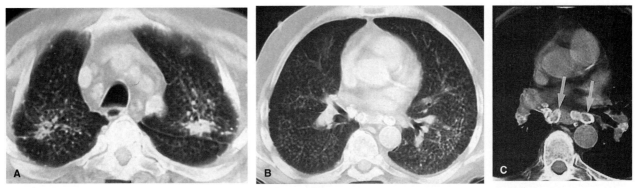

Figure 11-23

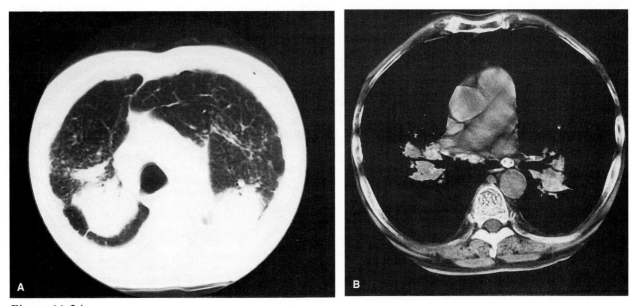

Figure 11-24

FIGURES 11-23 and 11-24

HRCT scans from two patients with silicosis show conglomerate masses, also called progressive massive fibrosis, in the upper lungs indicating complicated silicosis (coal-worker's pneumoconiosis has a similar appearance). Conglomerate masses arise from a coalescence of silicotic nodules and tend to develop in the midportion or periphery of the upper lobes and migrate toward the hila. Paracicatricial emphysema usually develops between the conglomerate mass and the pleura. Also, note the typical eggshell calcification of mediastinal nodes (*arrows*). Eggshell calcification may also be seen in sarcoidosis (see Fig. 11-1).

Alveolar microlithiasis

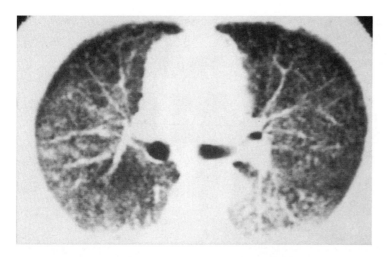

FIGURE 11-25

CT scan from a patient with alveolar microlithiasis shows diffuse, bilateral tiny calcified nodules. Differential diagnostic considerations include metastatic calcification, aspiration of barium, talcosis, and silicosis. Alveolar microlithiasis is a very rare disease of unknown etiology, characterized by the accumulation of intra-alveolar microliths. Most patients with alveolar microlithiasis are asymptomatic until late in the disease, when pulmonary fibrosis can develop.

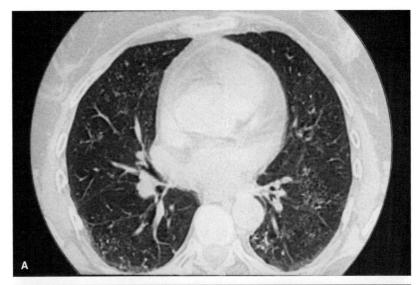

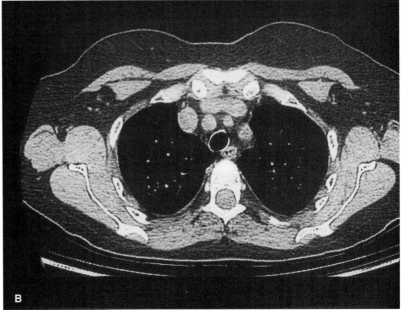

FIGURE 11-26

HRCT scans from a patient with chronic renal failure and secondary hyperparathyroidism show bilateral ill-defined lung nodules (A). These were calcified on the soft-tissue window settings (B). Findings are characteristic of metastatic calcification.

REFERENCES

1. Brauner MW, Grenier P, Mompoint D, Lenoir S. Pulmonary sarcoidosis: Evaluation with high-resolution CT. Radiology 1989; 172:467–471

2. Brauner MW, Lenoir S, Grenier P, Cluzel P, Battesti JP, Valeyre D. Pulmonary sarcoidosis: CT assessment of lesion reversibility. Radiology 1992; 182:349–354

3. Bergin CJ, Müller NL, Vedal S, Chan Yeung M. CT in silicosis: Correlation with plain films and pulmonary function tests. AJR 1986; 146:477–483

High-Resolution CT of the Chest: Comprehensive Atlas
by Eric J. Stern and Stephen J. Swensen,
Lippincott–Raven Publishers, Philadelphia © 1996.

Infectious Diseases
12

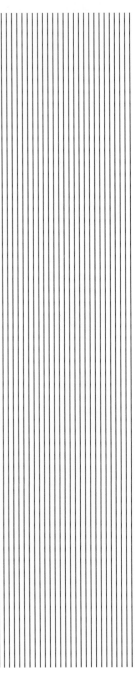

Fibrocavitary tuberculosis

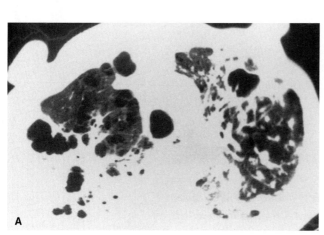
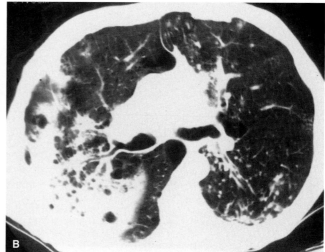

Figure 12-1

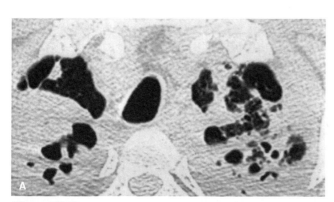
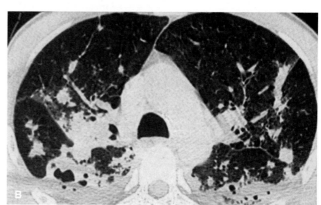

Figure 12-2

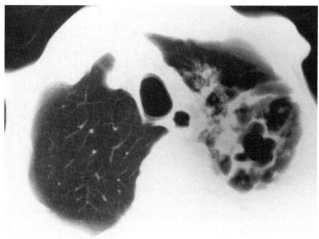
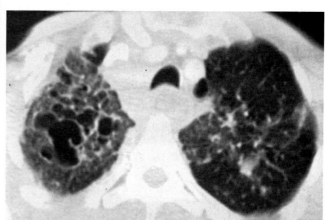

Figure 12-3

Figure 12-4

FIGURES 12-1, 12-2, 12-3, and 12-4

HRCT scans from four patients show typical manifestations of reactivation tuberculosis. There are extensive fibrocavitary changes in the lung apices of these patients. Multiple cavities with extensive cicatricial changes are common features that result in upper lobe volume loss, often with shift of the trachea to the ipsilateral side. Lymphadenopathy is not a common feature of reactivation tuberculosis. The organisms spread hematogenously to the lung apices during the primary tuberculous infection, where they can remain dormant for years before reactivating. Because *Mycobacterium tuberculosis* is an obligate aerobe, the high oxygen tensions in the upper lungs offer an ideal environment for these organisms to thrive. The presence of cavitation in reactivation tuberculosis is not in and of itself indicative of disease activity but should be considered indeterminate for activity. Comparison with old radiographs or CT scans is essential to determine disease stability.

Fibrocavitary tuberculosis—mycetoma

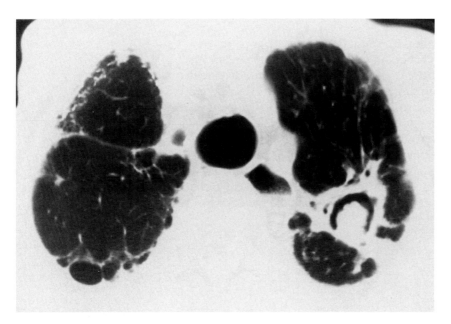

FIGURE 12-5

HRCT scan from a patient with fibrocavitary tuberculosis shows a rounded mass, in a dependent position, within a left upper lobe cavity. Note the surrounding fibrotic changes. Cavities of any etiology, but particularly tuberculous cavities, may become secondarily involved with saprophytic fungi, usually an *Aspergillus* species, resulting in mycetoma formation.

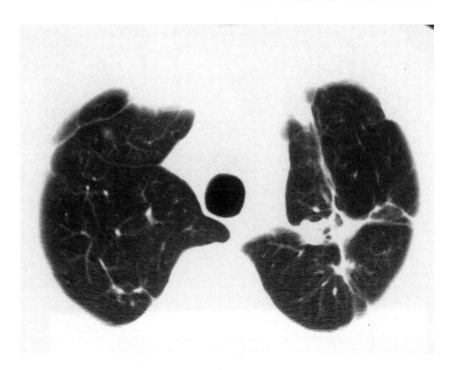

FIGURE 12-6

HRCT scan from a patient with a prior tuberculous infection shows fibronodular scarring in the left upper lobe. Dormant organisms can always be present, so without prior examinations disease activity should be considered indeterminate.

Endobronchial tuberculosis

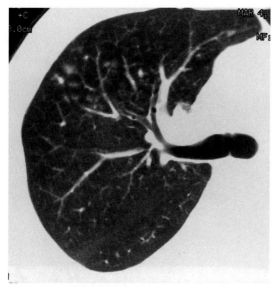

Figure 12-7

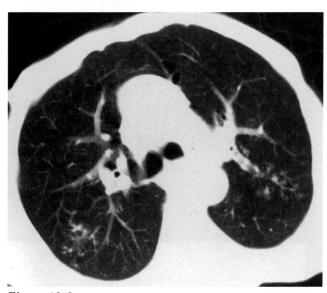

Figure 12-8

Figure 12-9

FIGURES 12-7, 12-8, and 12-9

CT scans from these three patients with sputum-positive tuberculosis show small, ill-defined peripheral acinar nodules grouped around small bronchovascular bundles; the grouping of these nodules suggests multiple abnormally filled acini within one or several secondary pulmonary lobules (see Chapter 2). This "tree-in-bud" appearance of active tuberculosis with endobronchial spread is characteristic but not pathognomonic of active tuberculosis. In the proper clinical setting, it is thought to be a reliable criterion for disease activity, distinct from old fibrotic lesions, as seen in Figure 12-6.[1] With appropriate medical therapy, these lesions often clear without residua. However, these nodules are nonspecific and may be seen with other processes, especially other granulomatous processes, such as atypical mycobacterial infection, fungal infection, sarcoidosis (Fig. 11-12), or even barium aspiration (Fig. 11-20).

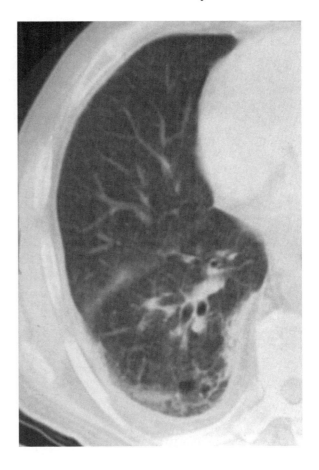

FIGURE 12-10

CT scan from this patient with tuberculosis shows innumerable diffuse miliary nodules. Miliary tuberculosis is usually a complication of primary tuberculosis, although it may result from reactivation of a latent infection. It represents hematogenous spread from the primary focus of infection. A similar miliary pattern may also be seen with sarcoidosis (Fig. 11-5), silicosis, fungal infections such as histoplasmosis (Figs. 12-29 through 12-32), coccidioidomycosis (Fig. 12-25), and rheumatoid lung disease (Fig. 8-19).

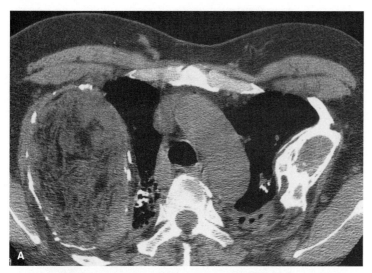

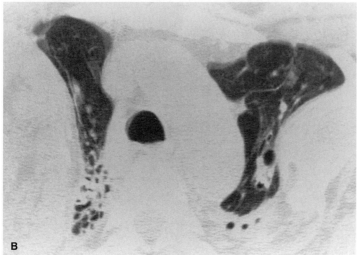

FIGURE 12-11

HRCT scan from a patient with prior treated tuberculosis shows a plombage with wax in the right hemithorax (oleothorax) and a thoracoplasty of the left hemithorax. Prior to the advent of antituberculous antibiotics, several different methods of therapy were used to treat tuberculosis. Most of these therapies revolved around putting the lung at rest and included serial iatrogenic pneumothoraces, thoracoplasty, and plombage; in the last treatment different materials such as lucite balls or wax were placed into the hemithorax. Note the extensive upper lobe scarring and bronchiectasis as residua of tuberculous infection, radiographically indeterminate for disease activity.

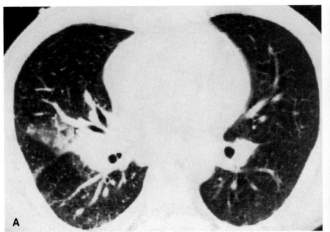
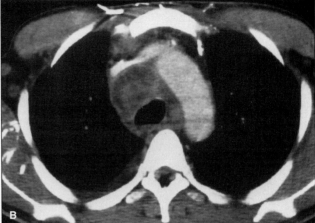

Figure 12-12

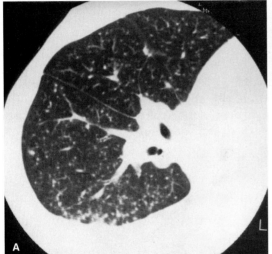
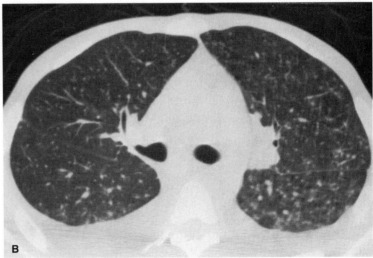

Figure 12-13

FIGURES 12-12 and 12-13

HRCT scans from two immunocompromised patients with human immunodeficiency virus (HIV) infection show parenchymal consolidation and adenopathy (Fig. 12-12*A, B*), miliary nodules, and pleural effusions from disseminated infection (Fig. 12-13*A, B*). The presentation of tuberculosis in patients with HIV infection depends on the extent of immune compromise. When the patient has a relatively normal immune system, tuberculous infection resembles that in the non–HIV-infected individual. As the immune system is compromised, tuberculous infection resembles that of primary tuberculosis, with consolidation and adenopathy or hematogenous dissemination, even though the disease is usually a reactivation of latent organisms.

Disseminated tuberculosis

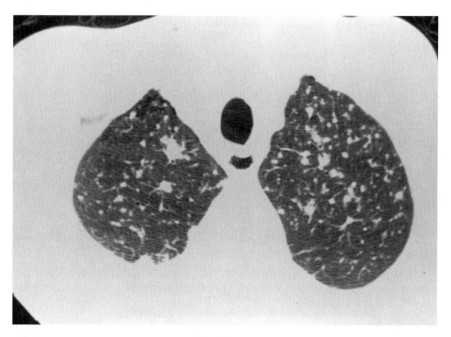

FIGURE 12-14

HRCT scan from this patient with AIDS shows multiple, ill-defined nodules throughout the lungs. This ill-defined nodular appearance is most suggestive of a granulomatous process, in this case, disseminated tuberculosis. The differential diagnosis would include many other disseminated viral and fungal pathogens.

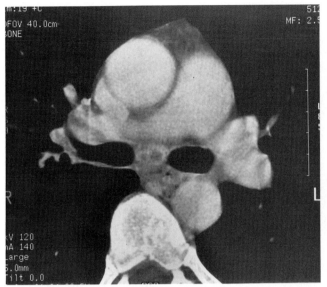

Figure 12-15

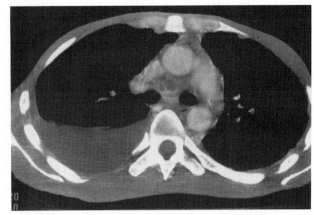

Figure 12-16

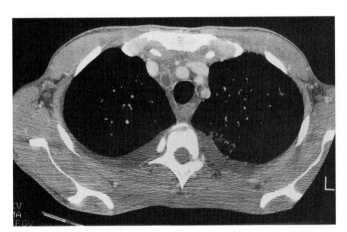

Figure 12-17

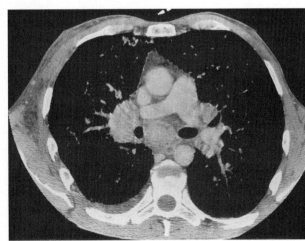

Figure 12-18

FIGURES 12-15, 12-16, 12-17, and 12-18

HRCT scans from these four immunocompromised patients with HIV-related tuberculosis show both peripheral enhancing necrotic lymph nodes and diffusely enhancing lymph nodes as part of the spectrum of adenopathy seen in HIV-related tuberculosis. This finding may also be seen in histoplasmosis or cryptococcosis but is less common with lymphoma or Kaposi's sarcoma.

Mycobacterium avium-intracellulare *complex*

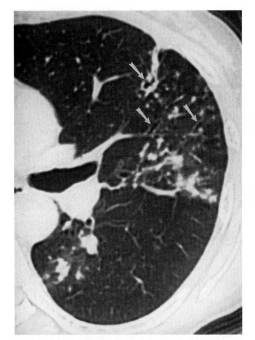

Figure 12-19

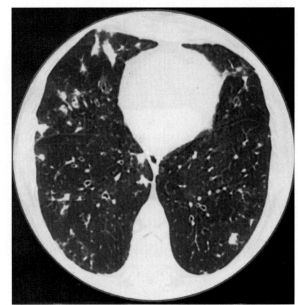

Figure 12-20

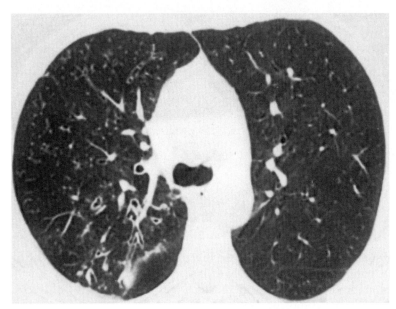

Figure 12-21

FIGURES 12-19, 12-20, and 12-21

HRCT scans from three patients with *Mycobacterium avium-intracellulare* complex infection show bronchiectasis with associated small nodular opacities. This combination of findings is a common manifestation of nontuberculous mycobacterial infection, often with *Mycobacterium avium-intracellulare* complex. Among immunocompetent patients, this disease appears to be more prevalent in the lower lobes of older women.

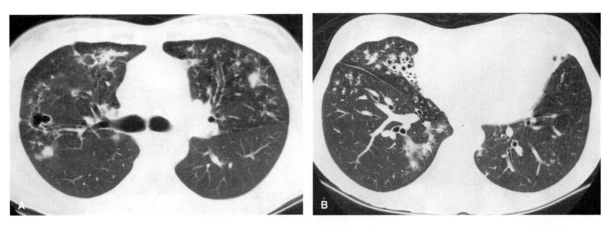

FIGURE 12-22

HRCT scans from this patient with AIDS and *Mycobacterium avium-intracellulare* complex infection show bronchiectasis with associated small nodular opacities; these manifestations are similar to those found in the immunocompetent host.

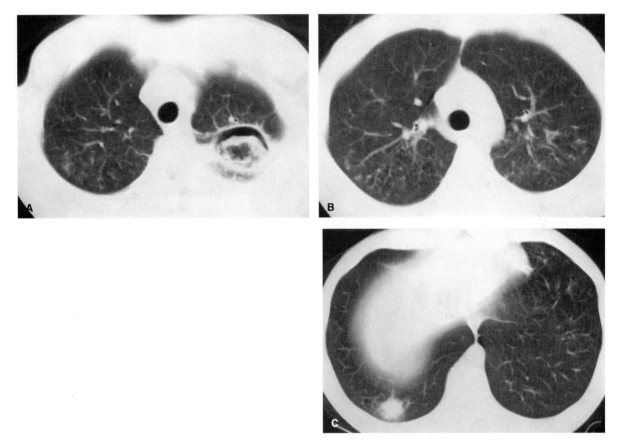

FIGURE 12-23

HRCT scans from this patient with AIDS and *Mycobacterium avium-intracellulare* complex infection show small, ill-defined peripheral nodules grouped around bronchovascular bundles, a large left upper lobe cavity with a mycetoma (A), and an ill-defined mass in the right lower lobe (C).

Mycobacterium avium-intracellulare *complex (continued)*

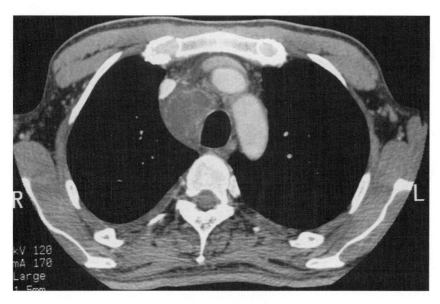

FIGURE 12-24

CT scan from this patient with AIDS and *Mycobacterium avium-intracellulare* complex infection shows an enlarged, necrotic, peripherally enhancing lymph node, which suggests a mycobacterial infection such as tuberculosis or *Mycobacterium avium-intracellulare* complex.

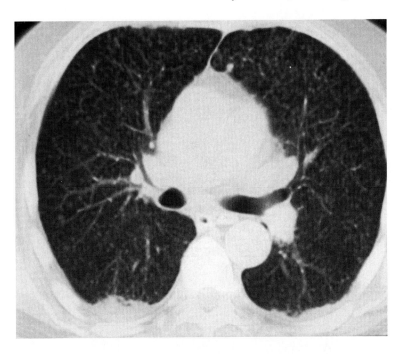

FIGURE 12-25

HRCT scan from this patient with coccidioidomycosis shows diffuse miliary (1 to 4 mm diameter) nodules. A diffuse miliary pattern is usually produced by a hematogenous process such as can be seen with the disseminated granulomatous infections such as tuberculosis (Fig. 12-10), histoplasmosis (Figs. 12-29 through 12-32), or metastatic disease.

Cavitary coccidioidomycosis

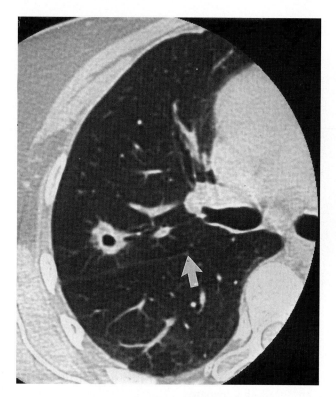

FIGURE 12-26

HRCT scan from this patient with coccidioidomycosis shows a 2.5 cm spiculated, cavitary nodule in the posterior segment of the right upper lobe. Spiculation is a sign that is usually more indicative of malignancy but can occur secondary to inflammatory processes, as in this case. Incidental note is made of an incomplete right major fissure (*arrow*) (see Fig. 2-7).

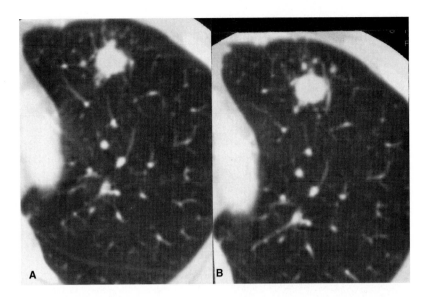

FIGURE 12-27

CT scans show a 1.5 cm noncalcified nodule in the left upper lobe. There are several tiny satellite nodules. Although nonspecific, this finding is indicative of a granulomatous as opposed to a neoplastic process, in this case due to *Histoplasma* granuloma.

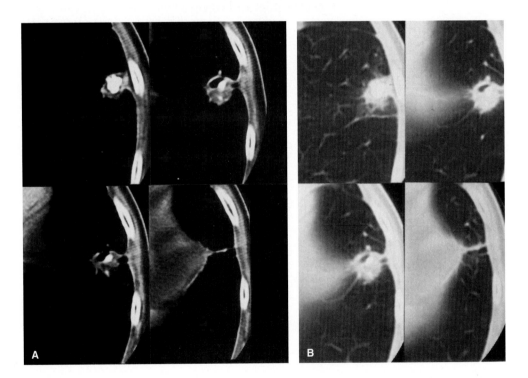

FIGURE 12-28

CT scans show a 2.5 cm spiculated, cavitary nodule with eccentric calcification and a pleural tail. CT findings are indeterminate but worrisome for scar carcinoma arising adjacent to a calcified granuloma. Video thoracoscopic biopsy showed the nodule to be a histoplasmosis caseating granuloma.

Disseminated histoplasmosis

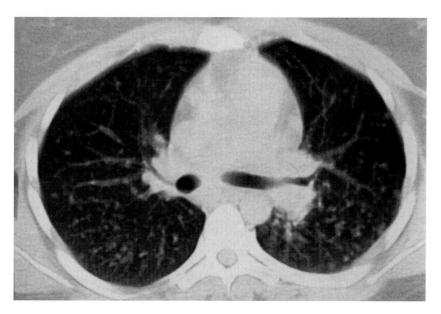

FIGURE 12-29

CT scan from an immunocompetent patient with acute histoplasmosis secondary to an overwhelming respiratory exposure to fungi. Disseminated disease in this case was not caused by hematogenous (miliary) spread (see Figs. 12-30 through 12-32).

Figure 12-30

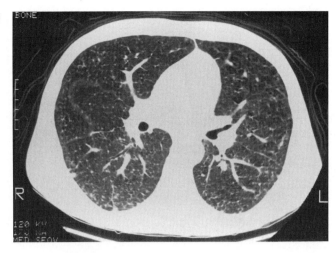

Figure 12-31

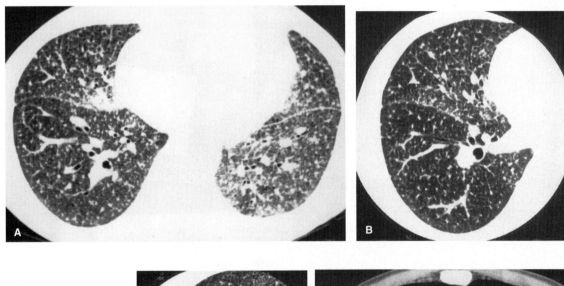

Figure 12-32

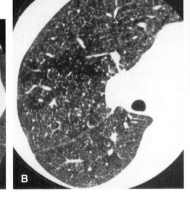
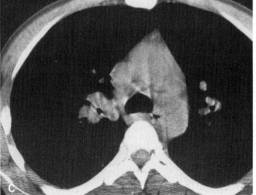

FIGURES 12-30, 12-31, and 12-32

HRCT scans from three patients with AIDS and histoplasmosis show typical miliary nodules throughout the lungs. In AIDS patients with histoplasmosis there is nearly always disseminated disease at presentation. In Figure 12-32C, note the associated right hilar adenopathy.

Septic pulmonary emboli

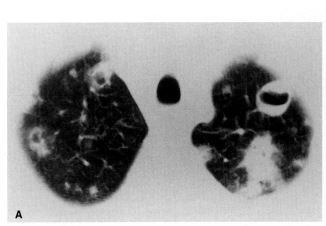

Upper lung zone

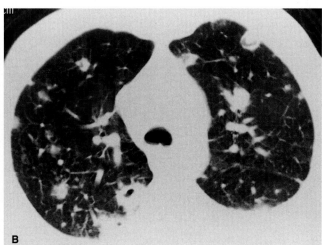

Middle lung zone

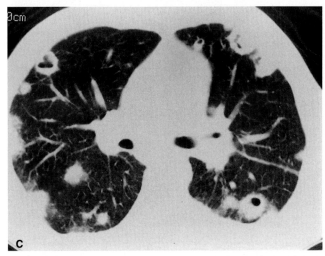

Lower lung zone

FIGURE 12-33

CT scans through the upper, middle, and lower lungs in a patient with septic emboli show multiple peripheral nodules and wedge-shaped opacities, many of which have cavities, scattered throughout the lungs. Some of these septic emboli have a "feeding vessel," suggesting their hematogenous etiology.[2] Wegener's granulomatosis (Figs. 10-25 through 10-27) and cavitary metastases (Fig. 10-13) can have a similar appearance.

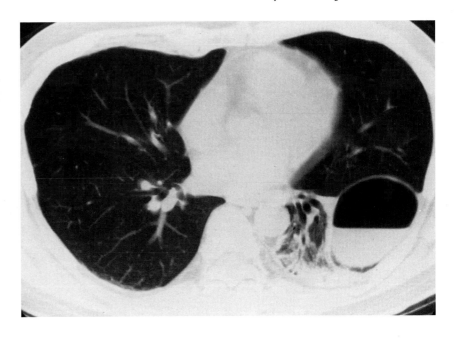

FIGURE 12-34

CT scan from a patient with a postinfectious pneumatocele shows a large, thin-walled cyst in the left lower lobe, an associated air-fluid level, and surrounding parenchymal consolidation. The CT scan was obtained 1 month into the course of pneumonia; the pneumatocele resolved completely within 4 months.

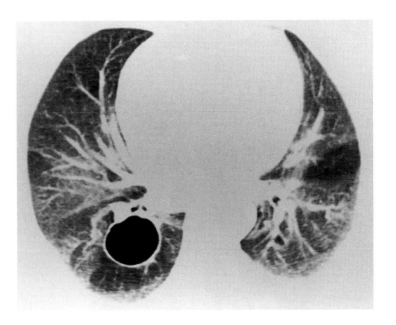

FIGURE 12-35

CT scan from a patient with a postinfectious pneumatocele shows a large, thin-walled cyst in the right lower lobe. This pneumatocele had not resolved 1 year after the onset of pneumonia; the patient was asymptomatic. Note the surrounding lucent lung consistent with mild air trapping.

Early bronchopneumonia

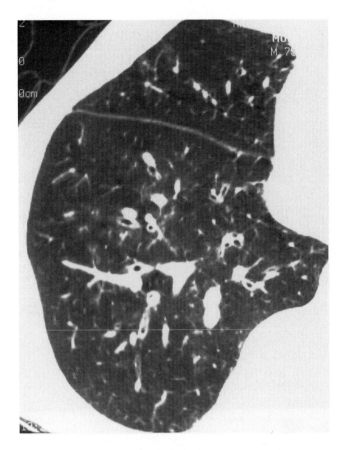

FIGURE 12-36

HRCT scan shows hazy ground-glass opacity around the lower lobe subsegmental bronchovascular bundles. This nonspecific finding (not evident on the chest radiograph) in this case represents an early bronchopneumonia that blossomed into a typical lobar pneumonia the following day.

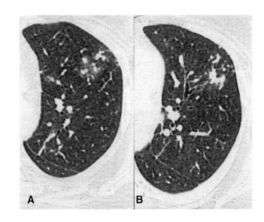

FIGURE 12-37

HRCT scan shows a nodular infiltrate in the left upper lobe. Directly adjacent to the solid components of these nodules is a ground-glass infiltrate or "halo." These findings in an immunocompromised host suggest that the most likely diagnosis is a fungal infection, particularly invasive aspergillosis, as in this case. Kaposi's sarcoma or an angioinvasive tumor can have a similar appearance.

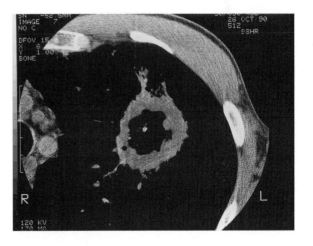

FIGURE 12-38

HRCT scan in an immunocompromised patient with invasive pulmonary aspergillosis shows a cavitary lung mass. Note the thick, irregular wall of the mass. Invasive pulmonary aspergillosis is not an infrequent abnormality in the immunocompromised host. Typical HRCT findings of invasive pulmonary aspergillosis early in the course of infection are single or multiple inflammatory nodules or masslike infiltrates representing bronchopneumonia. Air crescent formation has been reported to be highly suggestive of invasive pulmonary aspergillosis, but this is a late radiographic sign. Also early in the course of infection, a ground-glass–like halo around areas of consolidation may be seen;[3] this is a nonspecific sign that, in the case of fungal infection, corresponds to a central fungal nodule surrounded by a rim of coagulative necrosis.[4]

Allergic bronchopulmonary aspergillosis

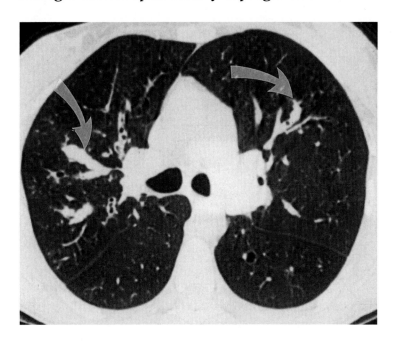

FIGURE 12-39

HRCT scan in a patient with allergic bronchopulmonary aspergillosis shows bilateral bronchiectatic airways with mucoid impactions (*arrows*). Allergic bronchopulmonary aspergillosis is not an infection per se, but a hyperimmune response to *Aspergillus* species. It results in excessive mucus production, impaction, and bronchiectasis. These patients are usually asthmatics and have elevated serum IgE levels.

REFERENCES

1. Im JG, Itoh H, Shim YS, et al. Pulmonary tuberculosis: CT findings—early active disease and sequential change with antituberculous therapy. Radiology 1993; 186:653–660

2. Kuhlman JE, Fishman EK, Teigen C. Pulmonary septic emboli: Diagnosis with CT. Radiology 1990; 174:211–213

3. Kuhlman JE, Fishman EK, Siegelman SS. Invasive pulmonary aspergillosis in acute leukemia: Characteristic findings on CT, the CT halo sign, and the role of CT in early diagnosis. Radiology 1985; 157:611–614

4. Hruban RH, Meziane MA, Zerhouni EA, Wheeler PS, Dumler JS, Hutchins GM. Radiologic-pathologic correlation of the CT halo sign in invasive pulmonary aspergillosis. J Comput Assist Tomogr 1987; 11:534–536

High-Resolution CT of the Chest: Comprehensive Atlas
by Eric J. Stern and Stephen J. Swensen,
Lippincott–Raven Publishers, Philadelphia © 1996.

Acquired Immunodeficiency Syndrome (AIDS)

13

Pneumocystis carinii *pneumonia*
Cytomegalovirus pneumonia
Varicella pneumonia
Cryptococcosis
Kaposi's sarcoma
Non-Hodgkin's lymphoma
Lymphoid interstitial pneumonia

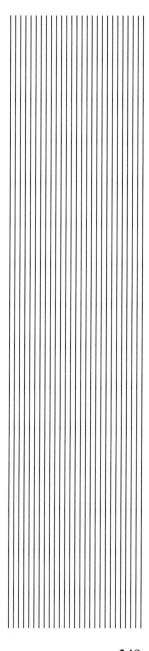

Pneumocystis carinii *pneumonia*

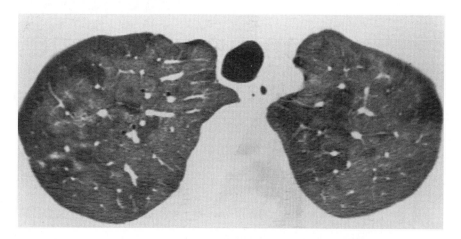

FIGURE 13-1

HRCT scan from this patient with AIDS and *Pneumocystis carinii* pneumonia (PCP) shows a predominantly ground-glass patchwork pattern of attenuation through which the vessels remain visible. This is the most common HRCT pattern of PCP. Other less common HRCT scan patterns of PCP are an interstitial pattern, nodules (sometimes called "PCPomas"), and upper lobe cavities and cystic spaces.[1] Occasional associated findings include pneumothorax, adenopathy, and pleural effusions (≤5%); these associated findings may be related to intercurrent disease.

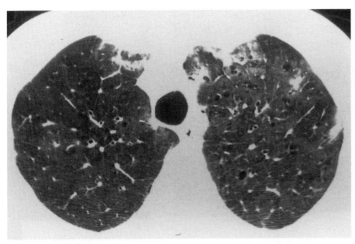

Figure 13-2

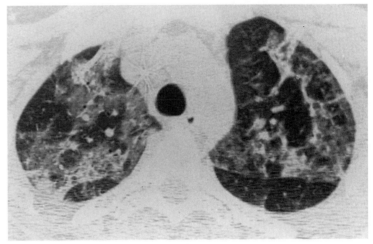

Figure 13-3

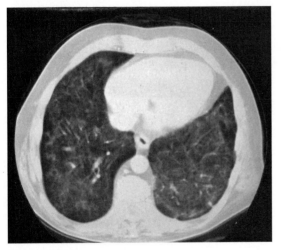

Figure 13-4

Figure 13-5

FIGURES 13-2, 13-3, 13-4, and 13-5

HRCT scans from these four patients with AIDS and PCP show typical diffuse but patchy ground-glass attenuation of PCP: mild (Figs. 13-2 and 13-3), moderate (Fig. 13-4), and severe disease (Fig. 13-5).

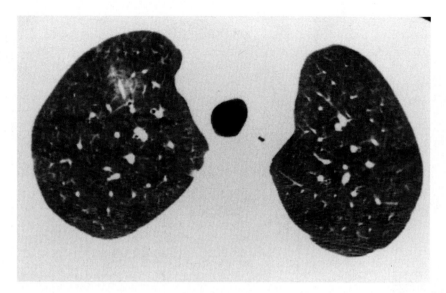

FIGURE 13-6

HRCT scan from a patient with AIDS and PCP shows a mixed pattern of nodular and ground-glass opacity as one of the variant appearances of this disease.

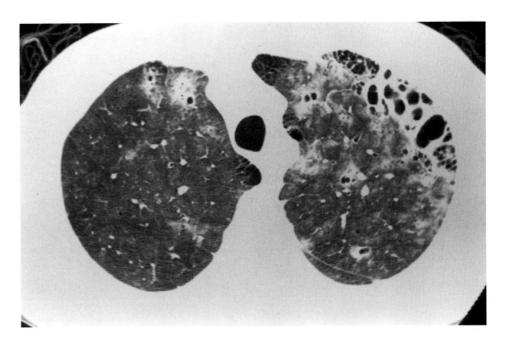

FIGURE 13-7

HRCT scan from a patient with AIDS and PCP shows both ground-glass attenuation and cystic lung disease. The *Pneumocystis carinii* organism can cause necrotizing, thin-walled, intraparenchymal cavities. These cysts are typically apical and sub-pleural, lined by fibrosis or alveolar parenchyma with little inflammation.[2] Cysts may appear in up to 40% of cases of PCP[1] and can either persist after clinical recovery or heal with no residua.

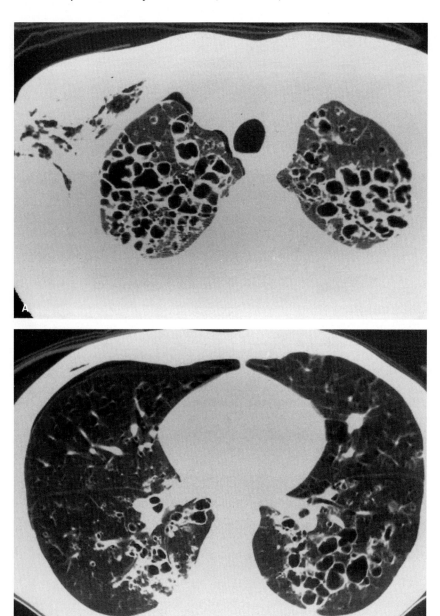

FIGURE 13-8

CT scans from a patient with AIDS and PCP show thin-walled pulmonary cystic lesions of PCP in both the upper (A) and the lower lobes (B). The upper lobe cysts are typical, whereas cystic disease secondary to PCP involving the lower lobes is less common.

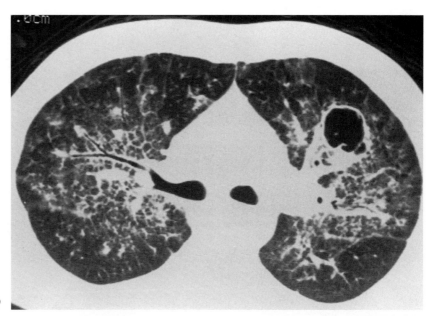

Figure 13-9

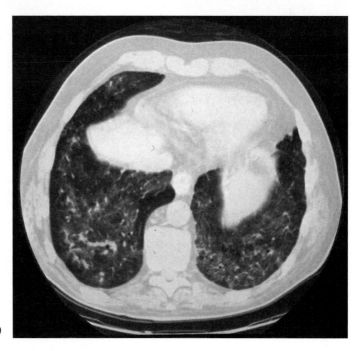

Figure 13-10

FIGURES 13-9 and 13-10

HRCT scans from two patients with AIDS and PCP show more of a reticular pattern than a ground-glass pattern. Note both fine and coarse reticular patterns. The reticular pattern seen in (Fig. 13-9), most apparent in the central perihilar regions, has a similar appearance to pulmonary alveolar proteinosis (see Figs. 2-22 and 2-23) and sarcoidosis (see Figs. 11-9 through 11-11).

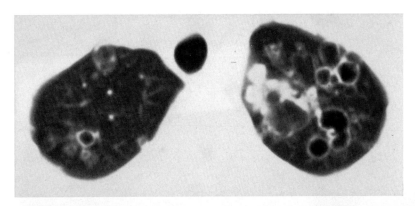

Figure 13-11

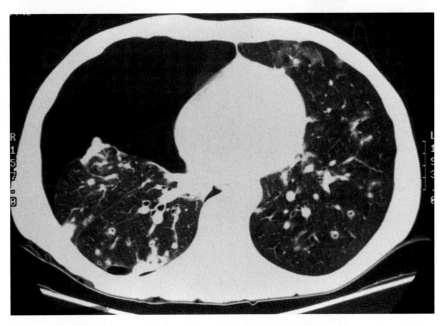

Figure 13-12

FIGURES 13-11 and 13-12

HRCT scans from two patients with AIDS and PCP show nodules or cystic nodules in both upper lobes. The patient in Fig. 13-12 has a right pneumothorax, a common complication resulting from the cystic changes of PCP.

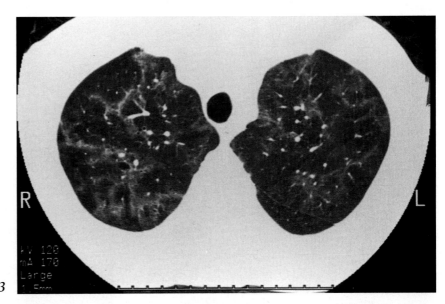

Figure 13-13

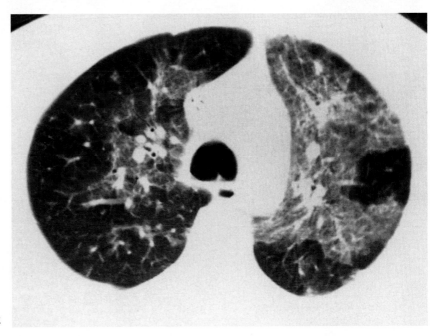

Figure 13-14

FIGURES 13-13 and 13-14

HRCT scans from two patients with AIDS and PCP highlight the variety of appearances that can be seen, including a nonlobular, nonsegmental pattern (Fig. 13-13) and a predominantly mosaic asymmetric pattern of ground-glass opacity (Fig. 13-14).

Cytomegalovirus pneumonia

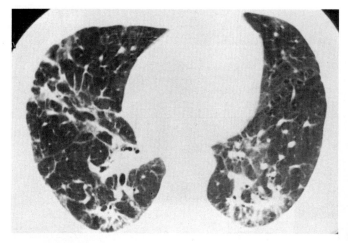

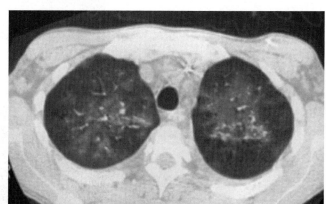

Figure 13-15

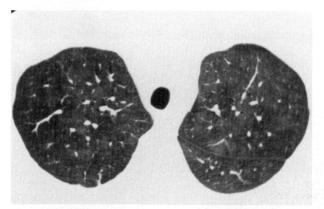

Figure 13-16

Figure 13-17

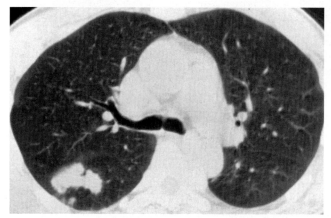

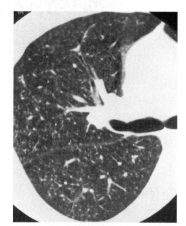

Figure 13-18

Figure 13-19

FIGURES 13-15, 13-16, 13-17, 13-18, and 13-19

HRCT scans from these five patients with AIDS show the spectrum of disease produced by pulmonary Cytomegalovirus infection. The most common CT findings are of a nonspecific mixed alveolar and interstitial disease (Fig. 13-15).[4] Ground-glass opacities (Figs. 13-16 and 13-17), masses (Fig. 13-18), and a miliary pattern (Fig. 13-19) can also be seen, all of which are nonspecific; biopsy is essential for accurate diagnosis.

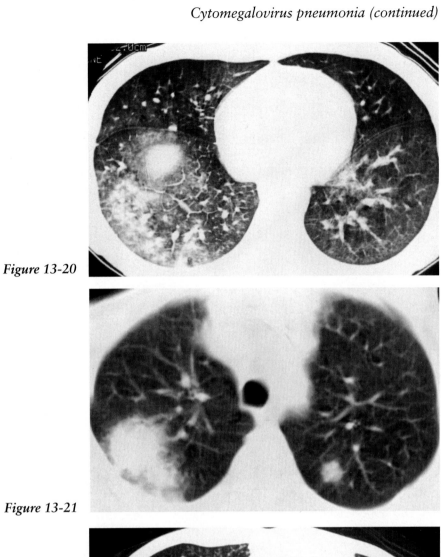

Figure 13-20

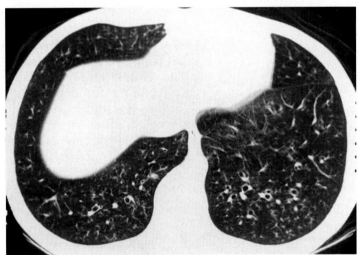

Figure 13-21

Figure 13-22

FIGURES 13-20, 13-21, and 13-22

CT scans from these three patients with AIDS again show the spectrum of pulmonary disease produced by Cytomegalovirus infection. Note the parenchymal consolidation (Fig. 13-20), discrete masses (Fig. 13-21), and bronchiectasis (Fig. 13-22).

Varicella pneumonia

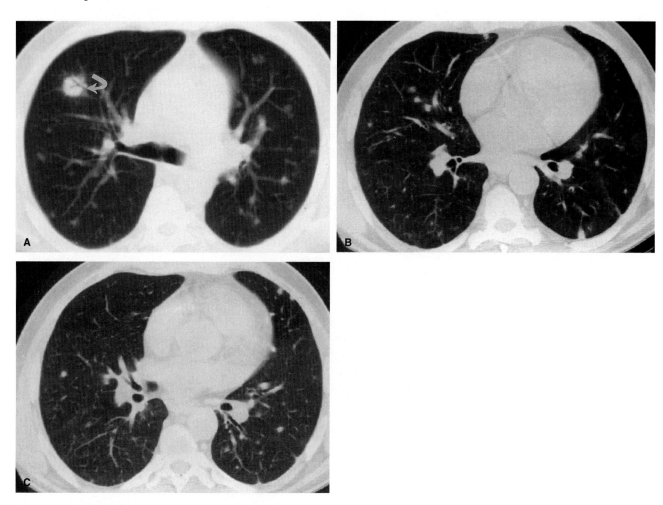

FIGURE 13-23

HRCT scans from this patient with AIDS and varicella pneumonia show multiple and fairly well-defined peripheral nodules of various sizes, the largest of which contains air bronchograms (*arrow*). These findings are nonspecific and may represent the presence of a number of pathogens or neoplasms.

Varicella zoster virus is one of the Herpesviruses (the others are Cytomegalovirus, Epstein-Barr virus, Herpes simplex virus, and Herpes virus-6). Varicella zoster is an unusual infection in patients with AIDS and may be either a primary or a co-pathogen.

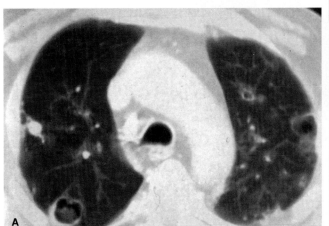

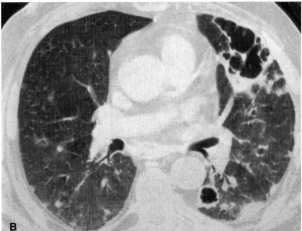

Figure 13-24

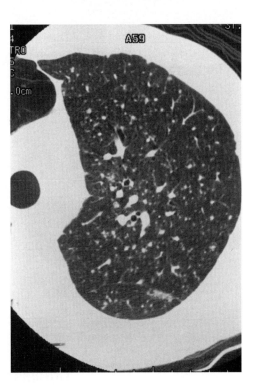

Figure 13-25

FIGURES 13-24 and 13-25

CT scans from two patients with AIDS and pulmonary cryptococcosis show numerous bilateral, cavitary, thick and irregularly walled nodules and focal infiltrates (Fig. 13-24*A, B*) and miliary nodules (Fig. 13-25).

Cryptococcus neoformans is a ubiquitous soil fungus that rarely causes lung disease in hosts with a normal immune system; the most common pulmonary fungal infection in patients with AIDS is due to *C. neoformans*. As shown above, common CT findings of cryptococcal lung infection are poorly marginated nodules or masses and diffuse scattered miliary nodules. Associated adenopathy, pleural effusions, and cavitation are uncommon.

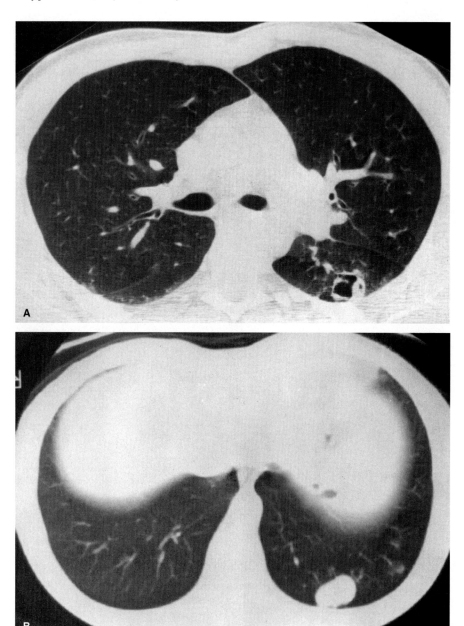

FIGURE 13-26

HRCT scans from a patient with AIDS and pulmonary cryptococcosis show both solid and cavitary masses. The HRCT pattern of cryptococcal pneumonia is usually nonspecific and may mimic other opportunistic infections or neoplasms; diagnosis requires biopsy or culture.

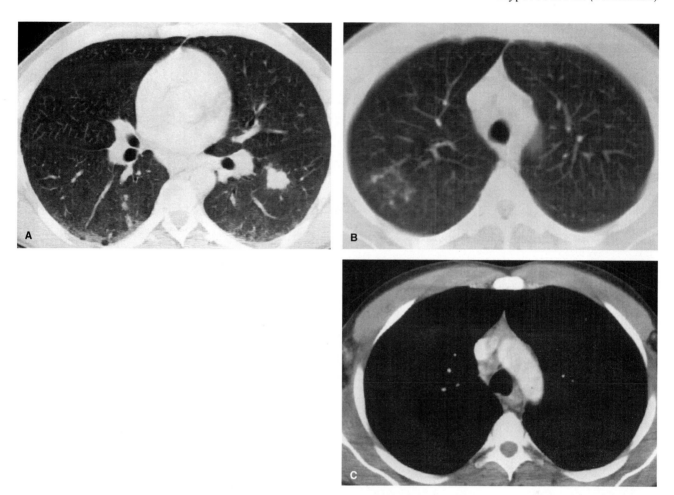

FIGURE 13-27

CT scans from this patient with AIDS and pulmonary cryptococcosis show, in addition to the more typical left lower lobe mass (A), multiple, clustered, ill-defined nodules in the right upper lobe (B). This is a nonspecific appearance but suggestive of a granulomatous process such as tuberculosis (see Figs. 12-7, 12-8, and 12-9), histoplasmosis, or, in this case, cryptococcosis. Also note the lymphadenopathy (C).

Kaposi's sarcoma

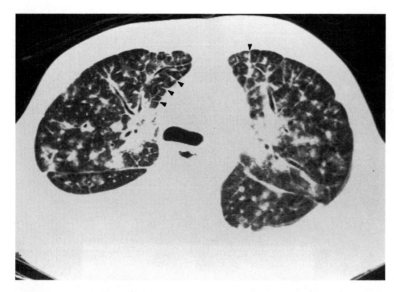

Figure 13-28

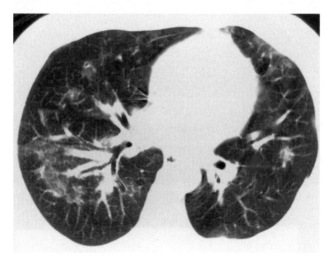

Figure 13-29   *Figure 13-30*

FIGURES 13-28, 13-29, and 13-30

HRCT scans from three patients with AIDS show characteristic opacities of Kaposi's sarcoma extending into the adjacent pulmonary parenchyma along the bronchovascular bundles. Figure 13-28 has an appearance similar to that of lymphangitic carcinomatosis (see Figs. 2-14 and 2-15). Note the interlobular septal thickening (*arrowheads*).

Kaposi's sarcoma and lymphoma are the most common forms of neoplastic disease encountered in patients with AIDS. Pulmonary involvement is fairly common with Kaposi's sarcoma, whereas lymphoma only rarely involves the lungs. HRCT can show shotty adenopathy, but true enlarged lymph nodes are unusual with Kaposi's sarcoma.[5]

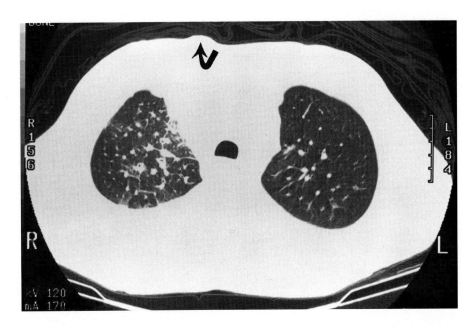

FIGURE 13-31

CT scan from this patient with AIDS shows moderate thickening of the right upper lobe bronchovascular structures and interlobular septa in this milder case of Kaposi's sarcoma. Note the skin lesions on the anterior chest wall (*arrow*).

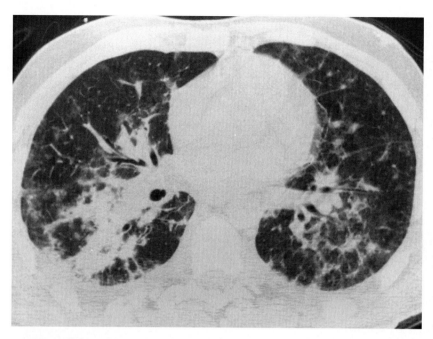

Figure 13-32

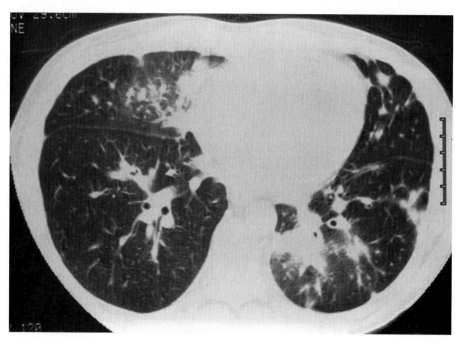

Figure 13-33

FIGURES 13-32 and 13-33

HRCT scans from two patients with AIDS show features of both Kaposi's sarcoma and PCP, a common scenario. Note both peribronchovascular thickening (Kaposi's sarcoma) and the patchy ground-glass attenuation (PCP).

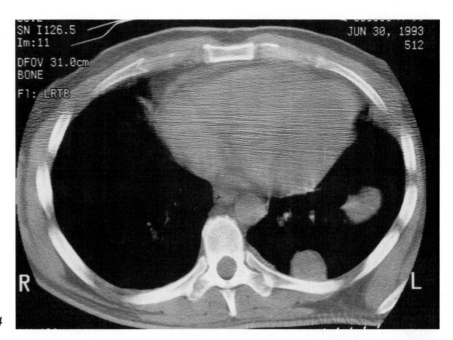

Figure 13-34

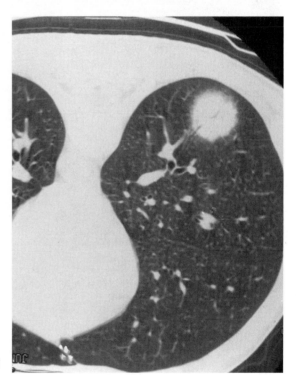

Figure 13-35

FIGURES 13-34 and 13-35

HRCT scans from two patients with AIDS and non-Hodgkins lymphoma show multiple nonspecific masses (Fig. 13-34) and a solitary nonspecific mass with a central air bronchogram (Fig. 13-35).

Lymphoid interstitial pneumonia

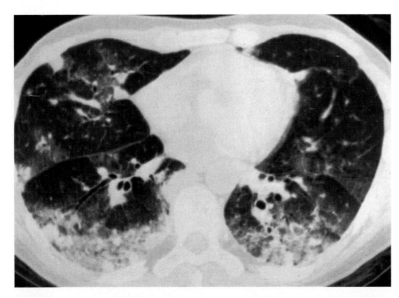

Figure 13-36

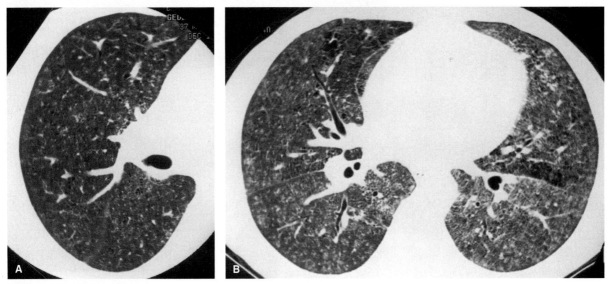

Figure 13-37

FIGURES 13-36 and 13-37

HRCT scans from two patients with AIDS and lymphoid interstitial pneumonia (LIP) show both nonspecific, patchy parenchymal consolidation (Fig. 13-36) and nonspecific, diffuse miliary nodules (Fig. 13-37).

LIP is a chronic condition that primarily affects adults and is becoming more common in patients with AIDS. LIP is an AIDS-defining illness in children with HIV infection. Histologically, mature lymphocytes infiltrate and expand the interstitium of the lung. Amyloid can also be deposited in the lung. LIP is considered a premalignant condition, converting to malignant lymphoma in up to 50% of non-AIDS patients.

REFERENCES

1. Kuhlman JE, Kavuru M, Fishman EK, Siegelman SS. *Pneumocystis carinii* pneumonia: Spectrum of parenchymal CT findings. Radiology 1990; 175:711–714

2. Feurestein IM, Archer A, Pluda JM, et al. Thin-walled cavities, cysts, and pneumothorax in *Pneumocystis carinii* pneumonia: Further observations with histopathologic correlation. Radiology 1990; 174:697–702

3. Moskovic E, Miller R, Pearson M. High resolution computed tomography of *Pneumocystis carinii* pneumonia in AIDS. Clin Radiol 1990; 42:239–243

4. Aafedt BC, Halvorsen RAJ, Tylen U, Hertz M. Cytomegalovirus pneumonia: Computed tomography findings. Can Assoc Radiol J 1990; 41:276–280

5. Naidich DP, Tarras M, Garay SM, Birnbaum B, Rybak BJ, Schinella R. Kaposi's sarcoma. CT-radiographic correlation. Chest 1989; 96:723–728

High-Resolution CT of the Chest: Comprehensive Atlas
by Eric J. Stern and Stephen J. Swensen,
Lippincott–Raven Publishers, Philadelphia © 1996.

Pitfalls and Artifacts
14

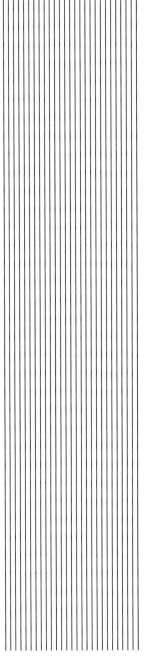

Effect of window settings on detection of emphysema
Effect of window settings on detection of air trapping
Effect of window settings on the appearance of pulmonary fibrosis
Effect of window settings on size of nodules
Effect of laser camera setting and window setting on image sharpness
Effect of supine and prone positions
Dependent lung density
Atelectasis
Unusual fissure position
Respiratory motion artifact
Respiratory motion artifact: Pseudobronchiectasis
Cardiac motion artifacts
Apparent ground-glass opacity

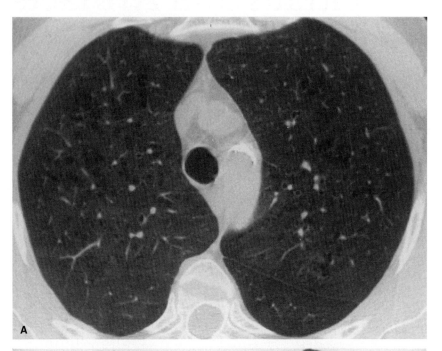

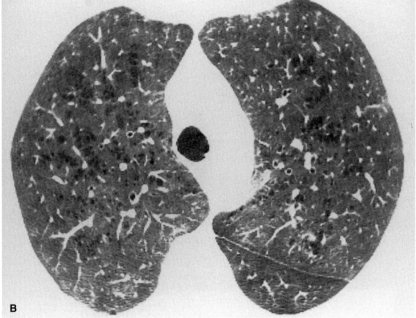

FIGURE 14-1

HRCT scan photographed at a window width of 2000 and a level of −600 (A) shows mild to moderate centrilobular emphysema. The use of this wider window width reduces contrast between the lung and emphysematous spaces, making the emphysema difficult to appreciate.

The same HRCT scan (B) photographed at a narrower window, width 500, level −800, has more favorable contrast between emphysematous spaces and normal lung parenchyma. This should not be considered a "routine lung window," but it does illustrate the effect of window settings on the detection of subtle contrast differences in the lung.

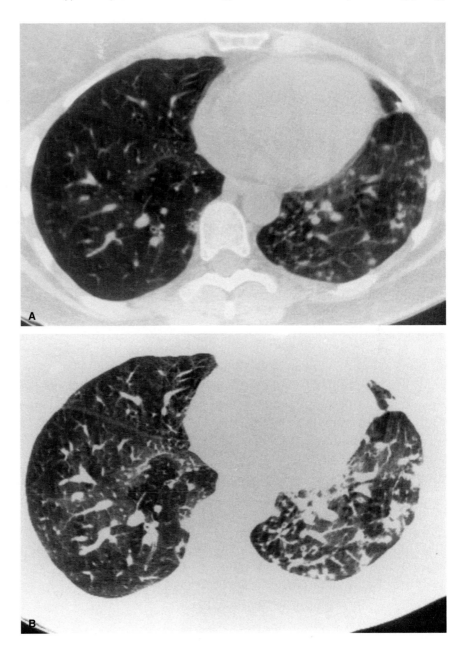

FIGURE 14-2

These expiratory HRCT scans, from this patient with bronchiectasis and air trapping, show the effect of window setting on the ability to visualize heterogeneous lung density. In (A), the wider window setting (width 2000 H and level −600 H) makes detection of air trapping (see Fig. 5-9) difficult. In (B), a narrower window setting (width 500 H and level −800 H) facilitates the detection of air trapping, showing that, on occasion, it is useful to tailor image photography to a particular patient or disease process to most advantageously display an abnormality.

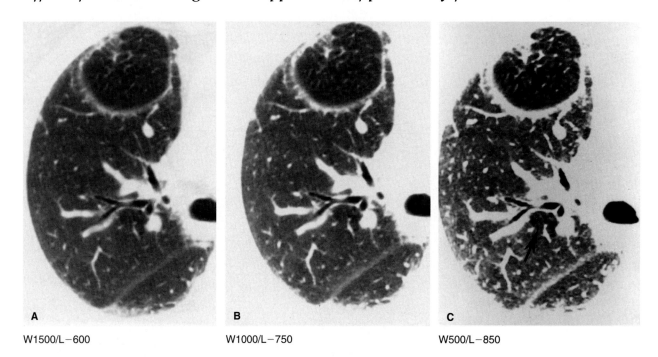

W1500/L−600   W1000/L−750   W500/L−850

FIGURE 14-3

HRCT scan from a patient with pulmonary fibrosis. Narrower window widths and lower (more negative) window levels can cause an artificial "blooming" in the size of small structures. Note the progressive apparent increase in thickness of the fissures, airway walls, and both large and small arteries and veins, from (A) through (C). At the same time that the blooming occurs, the accentuated windowing makes the emphysema more distinct (*arrow*). Although the use of narrow or wide windows can be helpful in selected cases, one should be aware of the attendant trade-offs and pitfalls.

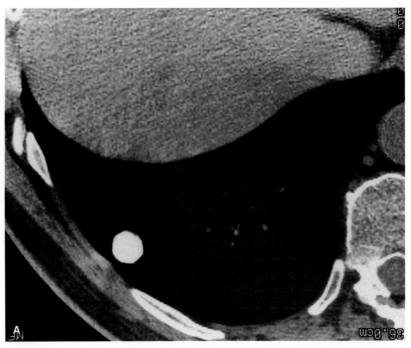

W500/L35

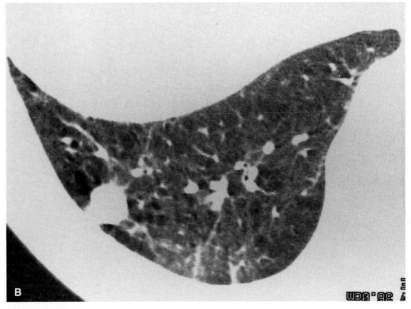

W600/L−880

FIGURE 14-4

CT scan from this patient shows a calcified solitary pulmonary nodule (A). The blooming effect is also evident with pulmonary nodules; the exaggerated negative window level falsely gives the impression that this calcified histoplasmoma is abutting the pleura (B). A routine lung window, W1500/L−700 (not shown) showed no pleural abutment.

Effect of laser camera setting and window settings on image sharpness

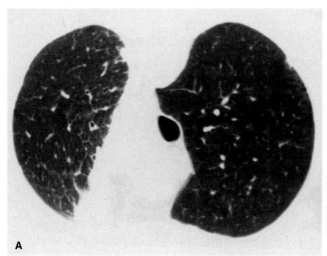

A

Smooth camera setting
W1500/L−700

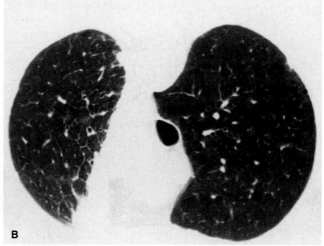

B

Sharp camera setting
W1500/L−700

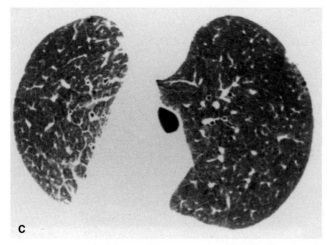

C

Smooth camera setting
W600/L−850

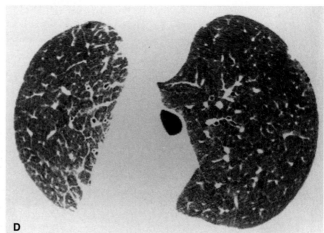

D

Sharp camera setting
W600/L−850

FIGURE 14-5

An HRCT scan in the prone position from a patient with lymphangitic carcinomatosis shows unilateral thickening of septal and bronchovascular structures. Not only can the CT parameters be optimized to produce a high-resolution image, but often laser camera sharpness also can be adjusted. Several commonly used laser camera manufacturers offer the choice of smooth (A and C) or sharp (B and D) image production, as shown. We prefer the sharp camera setting to optimize our resolution. Again, note the artificial blooming in size of small structures with the narrower setting in (C and D).

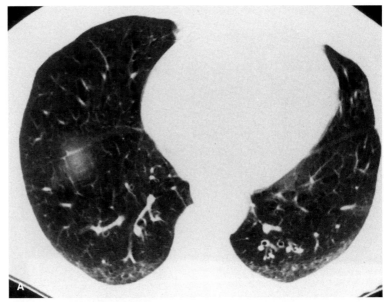

Supine

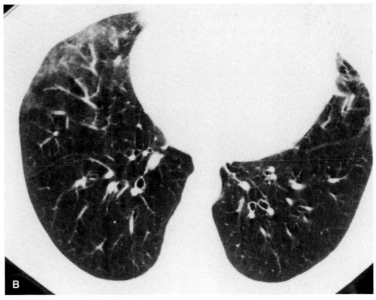

Prone

FIGURE 14-6

HRCT scan in (A) shows a zone of increased lung density in the dependent regions of the posterior lung bases. This is most often attributable to microatelectasis and other gravity-related changes. Unfortunately, this is very similar in appearance and distribution to the ground-glass opacity of many of the causes of pulmonary fibrosis (e.g., idiopathic pulmonary fibrosis, scleroderma, and asbestosis). So, in the clinical context of "rule out interstitial lung disease," to definitively state that these changes are caused by normal "dependent" lung attenuation or are secondary to pulmonary fibrosis/inflammation, the patient should be rescanned in the prone position. When the lung parenchyma is normal, the normal dependent lung density clears (B).

Dependent lung density

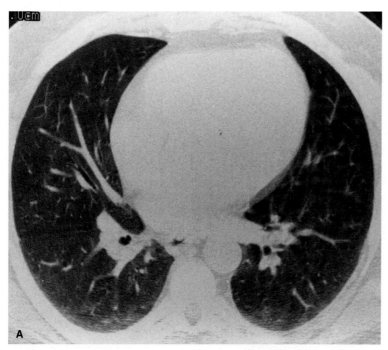

Supine

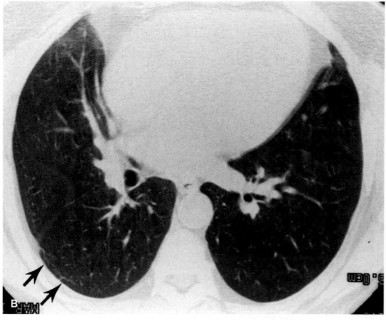

Prone

FIGURE 14-7

HRCT scan obtained in this patient with prior asbestos exposure shows "dependent lung opacity" (A) that did not completely clear upon repeat scanning in the prone position (B). In this case, dependent lung density was obscuring *mild* underlying fibrosis (*arrows*).

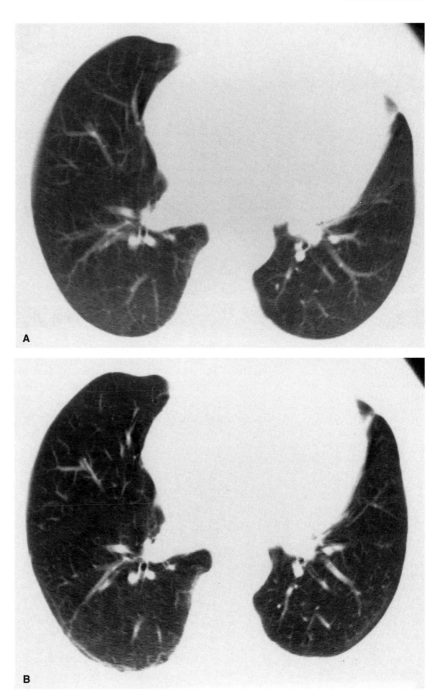

FIGURE 14-8

These two HRCT scans, at the same anatomic level from the same patient, were obtained just 15 minutes apart. Note the development of a subpleural line at the posterior right lung base and less so on the left (B). While a subpleural line in the proper clinical setting can represent confluent peribronchiolar fibrosis,[1] in this instance it was related to developing dependent atelectasis from prolonged supine positioning.

Unusual fissure position

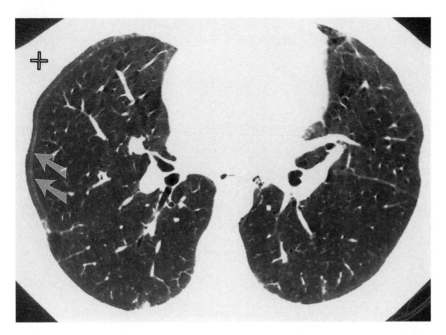

FIGURE 14-9

HRCT scan shows a thin subpleural line in a nondependent location (*arrows*). Occasionally, the minor fissure will be seen in such a cross-sectional plane as to mimic a fibrotic or atelectatic process. Viewing contiguous scan levels should easily clarify any uncertainty.

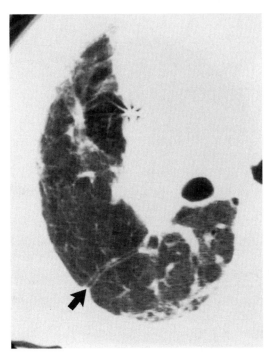

Figure 14-10

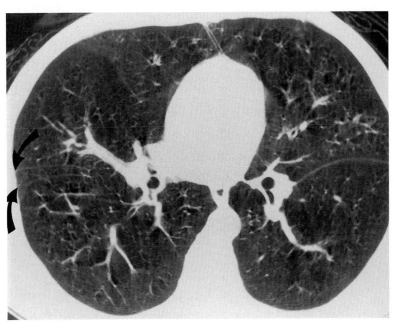

Figure 14-11

FIGURES 14-10 and 14-11

HRCT scans from two patients show an apparent double right major fissure (*arrows*).

   Patient breathing during CT scanning causes motion artifacts. Because HRCT shows the interlobar fissures so well, any significant breathing during scanning can cause a double fissure; as the CT detector array spins around a breathing patient, the fissure is imaged in two different positions.

Respiratory motion artifact: Pseudobronchiectasis

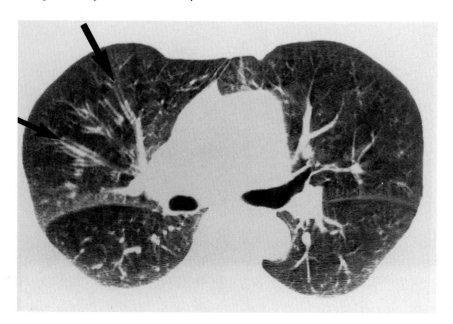

FIGURE 14-12

HRCT scan shows apparent dilated air-filled tubular structures that mimic bronchiectasis of the right middle lobe (*arrow*).

Pseudobronchiectasis occurs secondary to motion artifact of the airways. As the CT detector array spins around a breathing patient, the airways are imaged in two different positions.[2]

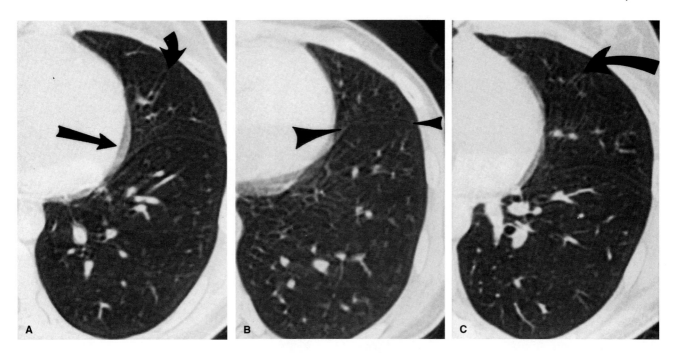

FIGURE 14-13

HRCT scans show motion artifacts in the lingula from left ventricular contractions during the 2-second scan time. Note a double left heart border (*arrow*, A) and double major fissure sign (*arrowheads*, B). The apparent dilated air-filled tubular structures that mimic the appearance of bronchiectasis (*curved arrows*, C) were caused by the same motion artifact that caused the double heart and major fissure signs.

Apparent ground-glass opacity

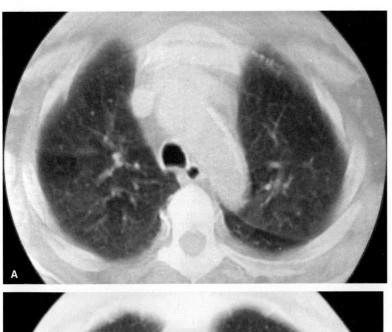

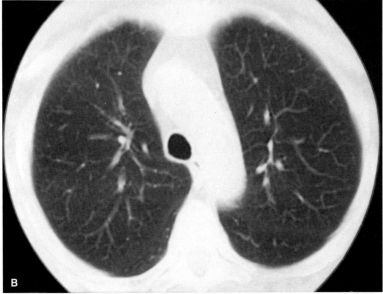

FIGURE 14-14

HRCT scans obtained accidentally at end-expiration may appear falsely abnormal, such as the apparent ground-glass opacity shown in this patient (A). Note that the tracheal shape is typical for end-inspiration (see Fig. 2-1). A full inspiration CT scan (B) was subsequently obtained at the same anatomic level and was normal.

REFERENCES

1. Akira M, Yokoyama K, Yamamoto S, et al. Early asbestosis: Evaluation with high-resolution CT. Radiology 1991; 178:409–416

2. Tarver RD, Conces DJJ, Godwin JD. Motion artifacts on CT simulate bronchiectasis. AJR 1988; 151:1117–1119

INDEX